# The Mediterranean Diet Cookbook

Over 100 Foolproof and Easy Mediterranean Recipes Using

European Measurements for Beginners (2022 edition)

Catharine White

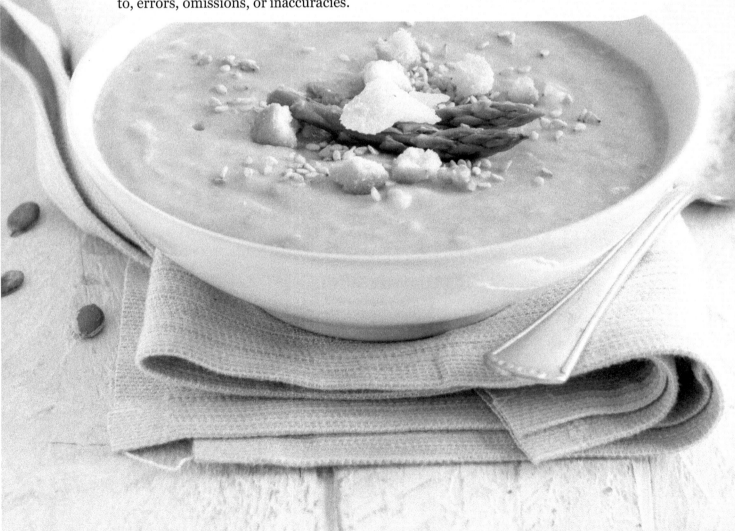

# Table of content

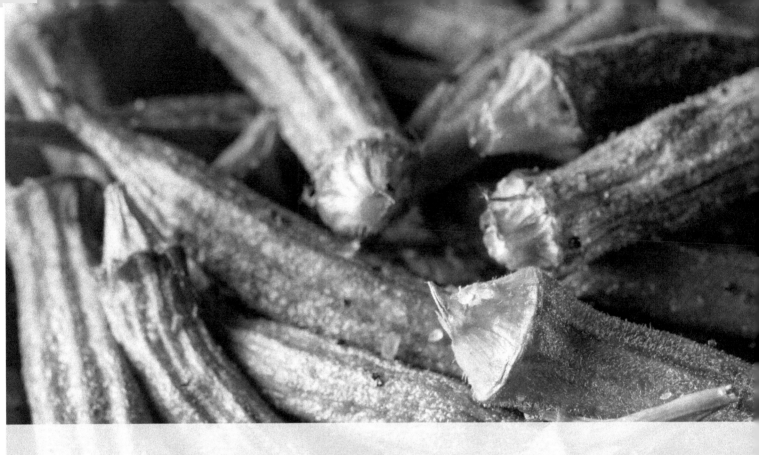

# INTRODUCTION

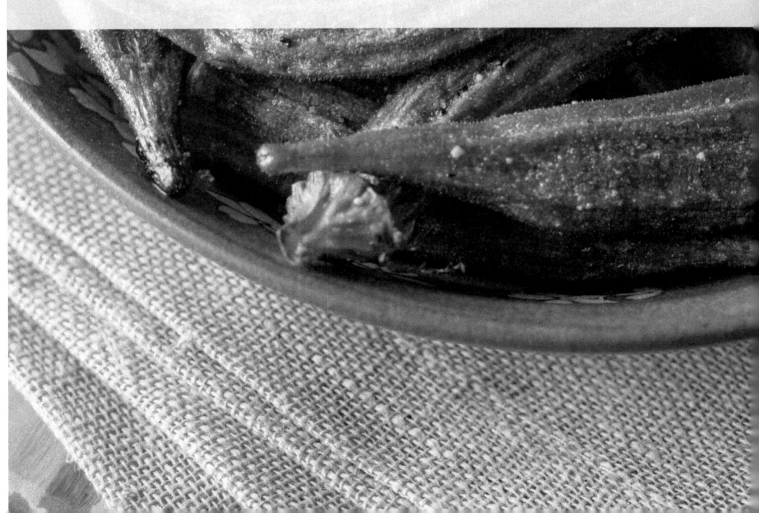

# INTRODUCTION

I have never been able to understand why the Mediterranean diet isn't more popular. I've heard of and tried all of the popular fad diets, but there hasn't been any success. In fact, they often made me feel worse physically, and the only thing many of them were designed to address was weightloss.

There is so much more to one's health than just a number on a scale. How about pain and aches? How about organ function? How about my mental health as well my physical health? Popular diets didn't focus on these things at all, and they were incredibly unsatisfying.

With these struggles in the back of my head, I did my research and found the Mediterranean diet.

This isn't like many of the other popular diets out there. Rather than being based on a specific aspect of nutritional science, the Mediterranean diet is a cultural practice.

The Mediterranean Sea is bordered by four European countries. Greece, Spain, France, and Italy all have access to a healthy supply of fish thanks to this geography. In addition to this, their climate allows for them to consume some of the same foods, but in a much different fashion.

This diet has been studied for years because of the incredible health benefits (Gunnars & Link, 2021). That was one of the first reasons I had been drawn to it. It doesn't just focus on your weight, like many other diets do.

The health benefits include brain health as well. I have always tried to use my brain to its maximum capacity. When other diets created a brain fog, I was left feeling extremely frustrated at the fact that I couldn't get more work done.
The Mediterranean diet also focuses heavily on fresh food sources.

One of my favorite parts of healthy eating has always been the fresh food. It tastes better and I do notice a difference in my body when I cook with these ingredients. It can take up some extra time during the week, but to save myself that trouble, I've set aside time to prepare meals on the weekends and that makes a difference (and I'm less tempted to go out for food, because what I need is already there).

Through many ways, the Mediterranean diet connects me to a culture of health and helps me feel great.

Once the basics are understood, it is very easy to follow!

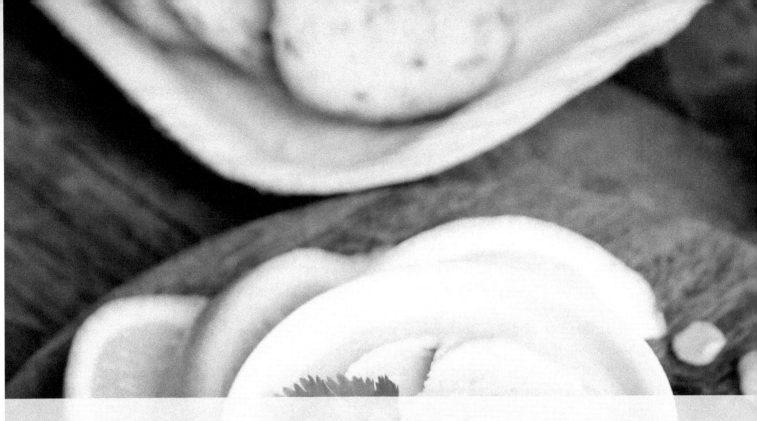

# CHAPTER 1: THE MEDITERRANEAN DIET AND IT'S CELEBRATION OF LIVE AND LIVING

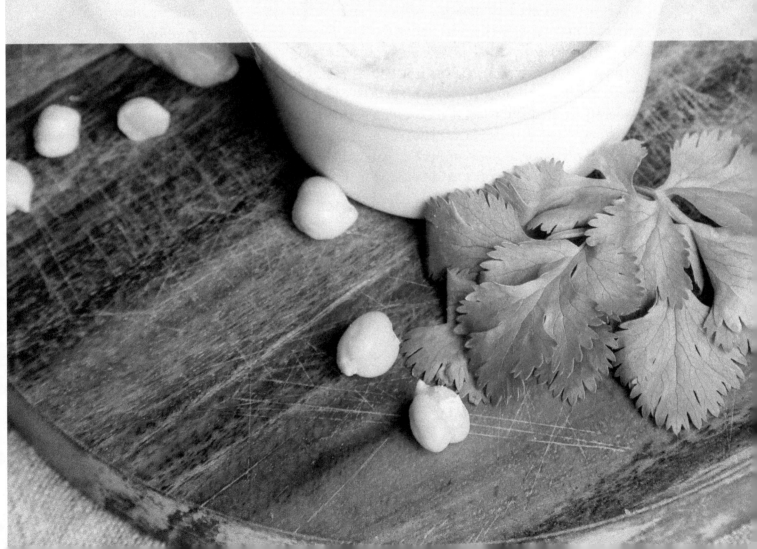

# Chapter 1: The Mediterranean Diet And It's Celebration Of Live And Living

## What is the Mediterranean Diet?

The Mediterranean diet is more of a cultural eating pattern than a full blown diet. It's origins come from Europe, particularly in the areas surrounding the Mediterranean Sea. It came to the attention of scientists because unlike the rest of the world, who tended to rely on similar foods (though in different quantities), this area wasn't facing epidemics of obesity, heart disease, diabetes, etc. This was jaw dropping to the era of people who were just discovering the role diet plays in overall health. The answer was found to be in the way they eat their food.

Unlike nearly every popular diet, the Mediterranean diet isn't centered around what you can't eat. Rather it focuses on how much of something you should eat, and the type of something you should eat. Due to the geography of the area, fish is a huge part of their diet. The climate of this area is also perfect for plant growth. Thanks to this, it's easier for those in this area to get a hold of fresh food than it is for them to get a hold of anything processed.

With the fresh fruits and vegetables being in easy reach, it makes up a major portion of the diet. What isn't so easy to get a hold of in this area is red meat. Because of that, it is severely limited. White meats are included much more in this diet, but not as often as fish.

Finally, if you are an alcohol lover, you will like this! The Mediterranean diet does include wine. Vineyards are not hard to come by in the Mediterranean region.

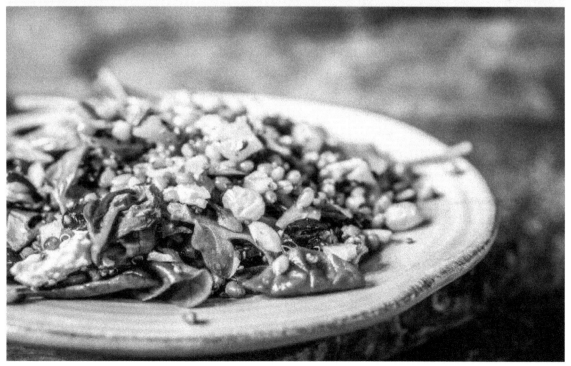

# Health Benefits of the Mediterranean Diet

One health benefit is that people in this area just seem to live longer. Their average age of death is higher because they don't have to worry about a lot of these common killers, which will often make up the top ten deaths in places like the United States.

One of these killers is heart disease. While it makes up a significant portion of deaths in the U.S., the Mediterranean diet aids the region due to it's low-fat content. There is evidence to suggest that it doesn't lead to nearly as much plaque build up in the arteries (Gunnars & Link, 2021).

It can have a great impact on your brain as well. Diseases such as Alzheimer's are much less common in those who follow this diet. It has also shown to help with overall brain function, with those who have been on it reporting that they can think and focus better (Gunnars & Link, 2021).

It protects us against diabetes. Much of the issues with diabetes come from highly processed foods and red meat that are not common in this area. The Mediterranean diet helps with inflammation and body function, and it can have positive effects on those who already have diabetes, and help others who are at risk avoid getting it altogether (Gunnars & Link, 2021).

Finally, there are certain cancers that are linked to diet. Liver cancer, for example, can stem from fatty liver which is a result of obesity. The Mediterranean diet protects against this.

# The Mediterranean Food Pyramid

Most culture-based diets do have a food pyramid that their diet is based on. This can be in common use around the country, or created by researchers as something that others scientists and curious individuals can reference.

The Mediterranean pyramid, in particular, has five slots. Four of these slots are dedicated to the food that should be consumed, and one is dedicated to the lifestyle. The outside of the food pyramid talks about two important liquids. Water is essential to the Mediterranean diet, and wine can be consumed in moderation.

Part of the Mediterranean diet involves its lifestyle. Physical activity and enjoying meals with others are a part of the diet. These things do actually affect how you eat and how food is metabolized in your body. Exercising engages your metabolism and changes how the food is going to be processed. Another aspect to consider is that eating with others has been proven to slow you down. You receive your fullness cue on time instead of when you have already eaten too much.

## *Foods to Eat*

First of all, fruit is very important! Fruit contains vital vitamins and minerals, and in this way of eating, you don't have to limit your consumption of them! Apples, oranges and other citruses, berries, peaches, mangoes, grapes, and more are all ready and waiting for you to make them a part of your diet. A little tip if you are craving something sweet is to have cut up fruit with you. Oftentimes, this will do the trick!

Vegetables, as you might imagine, are next on the list. Like fruit, vegetables also contain items that are vital to your health. Carrots, broccoli, spinach, lettuce, onions, and more are all now a major part of the diet. It's worth noting that the traditional Mediterranean diet also includes potatoes, but there will be a difference in the level of processing between their potatoes and ours. At the end of the day, if you want to enjoy a starchy treat, it's best to be able to name all of the ingredients it contains.

Whole grains are your next item in this section. This will mean a lot of substitution. Many breaded and carb items are filled with refined grains which are stripped of their minerals and tend to harm us more than they help us. Whole wheat bread, pasta, rice, and other breaded items are all fantastic options for some of your favorite carb rich dishes.

Olive oil is a huge part of the Mediterranean diet. Because this diet is low on processed items, dressings and cooking sprays are often out of the picture. However, olives grow naturally in this area, so it's understandable that they are such a big part of the diet. You can cook with it, add it to baked goods, make dips out of it, and use it in dressing. If you're bored of the same olive oil, specialty stores often carry a wide variety of flavors!

Up next are beans. Beans can be very filling and they are a great source of protein. With the Mediterranean diet, you won't be consuming as much meat, so these will become important!

We can't forget about nuts and seeds. A lot of vitamins and minerals will come from them, and some nuts even have protein!

Finally, there are herbs and spices. They add flavor to your food and they are full of rich vitamins and minerals for your body.

## *Foods to Eat in Moderation*

Anything listed above is something that should be a part of your diet every day. They take up a main portion of every meal. This next list, however, doesn't need to be included as often.

The most important ones on this list are fish, shellfish, and other seafood. You should be aiming to eat this at least two times a week. As discussed above, fish is a huge part of the Mediterranean diet. It provides a good source of healthy fat and protein. You should aim for fresh fish if you can!

Up next is poultry, which includes white meats such as chicken and turkey. These aren't nearly as hard on your heart as red meat tends to be. They still provide a great source of protein. You should be aiming for this anywhere from daily to weekly.

Up next are eggs. Like poultry items, eggs provide a great source of protein, but they aren't as important to the diet as items in the first category. You should also be aiming for a daily to weekly intake of this.

Next are the dairy products. This includes milk, cheese, and yogurt. Because these items have to go through some processing in order to be created, they aren't as involved in the diet, but they do contain some much needed nutrients (like Vitamin

D). They can also be a healthy source of fat in some cases. Try to aim for less processed options if possible and consume them anywhere from a daily to a weekly basis.

Finally, there is wine. Wine is a wonderful part of the Mediterranean diet, and is also something that should be consumed in moderation. That means something different to everyone. Whether you chose to have a single glass with a meal, or you chose to have a couple of drinks on the weekend with friends is up to you!

## Foods That Won't Be the Main Part of the Diet

The cool thing about the Mediterranean diet is that it doesn't really eliminate foods, instead it relies on amounts and limits.

The main thing for this will be processed foods. This is incredibly hard in countries like America, where everything does seem to have a lot of processing to it, but that processing is hurting us! In countries in the Mediterranean region, it's actually harder to get a hold of processed foods than it is to get a hold of regular food types. This may link to why their health seems to be a lot better as a population.

Steer away from processed options as much as your budget will allow. White breaded items can be swapped for whole grains (which is something to consume daily) at almost no cost. Aim for fresh fruits and vegetables if you can, but if you have budget concerns, or if you know they will go bad, start reading labels very carefully. These can provide clues as to what's been processed more.

Running along the line of processed foods are candy. These should only be consumed once a week at most. They are often highly processed and even when they aren't, they still contain things that aren't very good for us. If you like sweet things, make fruit a go-to in your diet. Dates are also a fantastic way to satisfy your sweet tooth. If you are still really craving that sugar, aim for dark chocolate. It still has many great minerals for you and it hasn't been nearly as processed.

Finally, there is red meat. Red meat has been linked to a variety of issues, including raised cholesterol, heart disease, obesity, blood pressure, diabetes, etc. No one is certain on why it seems to be causing us so much trouble, but everyone can agree that it is problematic and that cutting it down in our diet would help us. The Mediterranean region has never had the same access to red meat that we do and as a result, they are in better internal shape. You should be eating this, at most, weekly.

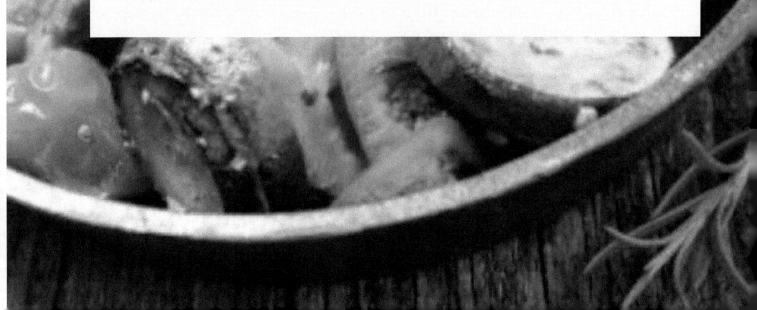

# Extra Virgin Olive Oil: The Core of the Mediterranean Diet

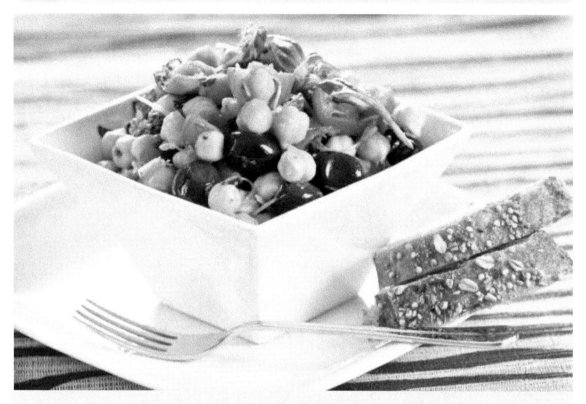

You may have heard before that substituting canola and vegetable oil with olive oil was a better choice. This is more than true!

Olive oil is a huge part of the Mediterranean diet. It can be cooked with, made into dips and dressings, and more. Olive oil is rich in the healthy fats you need, and finding the right kind means that you have an unprocessed oil to cook with.

When thinking of olive oil, you may just be thinking of the plain brand that ends up in every store, but there is more to it than that. If you know where to look, you can find specialty stores that sell olive oil in a variety of flavors with different processes to make them. Each one can add something amazing to your cooking!

If it is within your budget, I absolutely recommend trying out one of these speciality stores for your olive oil needs. They will have little to no processing, and their taste is impeccable.

If this isn't an option for you, then read the labels at your local grocery store carefully. Refined olive oil will be the most processed. Then there is virgin olive oil. Finally, anything labeled extra virgin olive oil will have the least amount of process, and it is associated with the most health benefits.

For extra virgin olive oil, you don't need to refrigerate it. With the other two, this is your best option. Do not store your olive oil next to the stove, as the heat can harm the potency of the oil and shorten its life. Keep it in a dark place and at room temperature. If you don't use it within a year, it may start to break down on you.

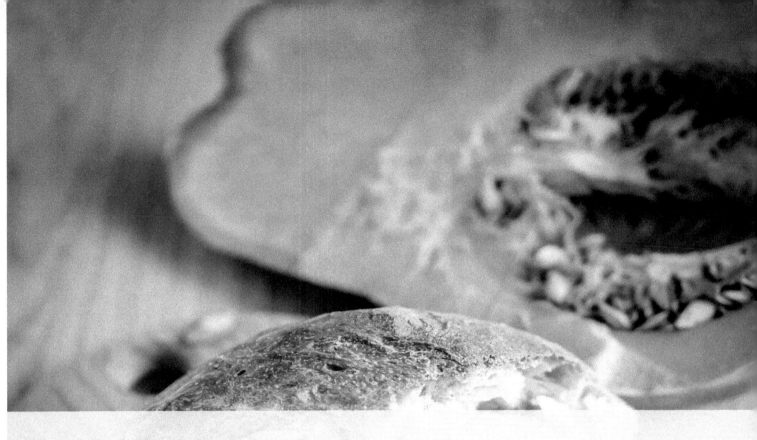

# CHAPTER 2: EIGHT STEPS TO GETTING STARTED

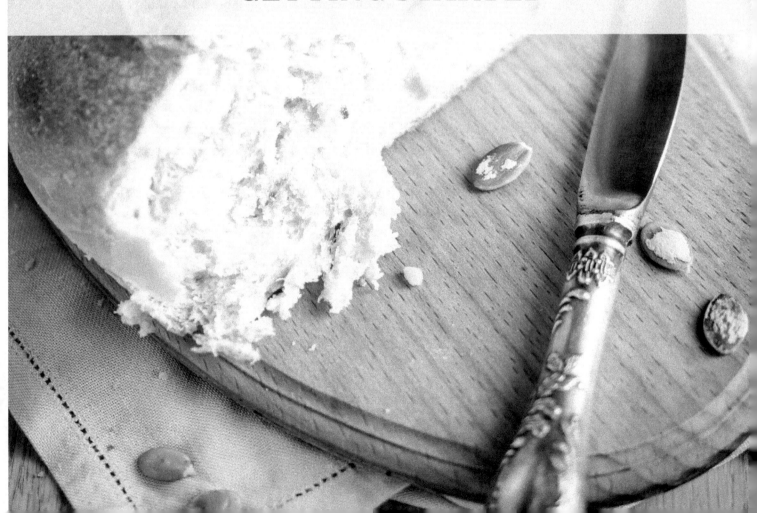

# Chapter 2: Eight Steps To Getting Started

### ❖ *Eat LOTS of Vegetables*

Vegetables are a major part of the Mediterranean diet. Technically, it's supposed to be a major part of all diets, but that isn't necessarily what happens. In many countries, fresh vegetables are often exalted, but they are expensive. When people think that frozen or canned items aren't good for them, they tend to leave without any vegetables. Whether it's fresh, frozen, or canned though, vegetables still have amazing benefits.

### ❖ *Change the Way You Think About Meat*

We are taught that protein is vital to our diet. It is stressed to us from a young age, and it often leaves us to believe that we should consume it in every meal. This isn't true.

Meat isn't the only protein source out there. Beans, nuts, wholegrains, and even dairy all contain what we need.
Furthermore, we don't need meat with every meal. Having a protein source in our diet once a day will satisfy our body's needs most of the time.

Meat, in particular, can be dangerous if over consumed. Heart disease and it's cousins, high cholesterol, high blood pressure, obesity, and diabetes, are all associated with over consumption of meat.

### ❖ *Enjoy Some Dairy Products*

People tend to over or under do it when it comes to dairy. If you eat too little, you aren't getting enough of the vitamins and minerals that contribute to bone growth. If you are eating too much then you run the same risk that you do when you eat too much meat.

The Mediterranean diet says to consume dairy on a daily to weekly basis. You don't need it every day, but you should be having it more than once a week.

### ❖ *Eat Seafood Twice a Week*

If your diet doesn't usually contain seafood, then this is a great place to start. Eating seafood twice a week can provide protein the same way meat can, and it provides you with healthy fats. Fresh fish is going to be your best bet if you can get a hold of it!

### ❖ *Cook a Vegetarian Meal One Night a Week*

How much do you consume when it comes to vegetables? With the Mediterranean diet, you should be consuming them with just about every meal. Cooking in a vegetarian manner allows you to do just that, and opens your mind to more possibilities. If you want to ensure your meal is filling, add beans or whole grains...or both!

## ❖ *Use Good Fats*

Olive oil! We are absolutely talking about olive oil here. Canola and other oils are extremely refined and can really hurt you in the long run. Olive oil, on the other hand, involves minimal processing and it is associated with great health benefits.

## ❖ *Switch to Whole Grains*

Even though other diets have tried to eliminate them, carbohydrates are important to your diet...it's the kind of carb that will matter. White grains are extremely processed and have had all of the vital vitamins and minerals removed from them. Whole grain options let you get your carbs in while also containing what your body needs!

## ❖ *Use Fresh Fruit to Satisfy Your Sweet Tooth*

Fresh fruit is incredibly sweet and full of nutrients. If you are like me and you get a sweet tooth, have something on hand from your local farmer's market! These won't contain processed additives that will do more harm than good, and they will make you feel better at the end of the day.

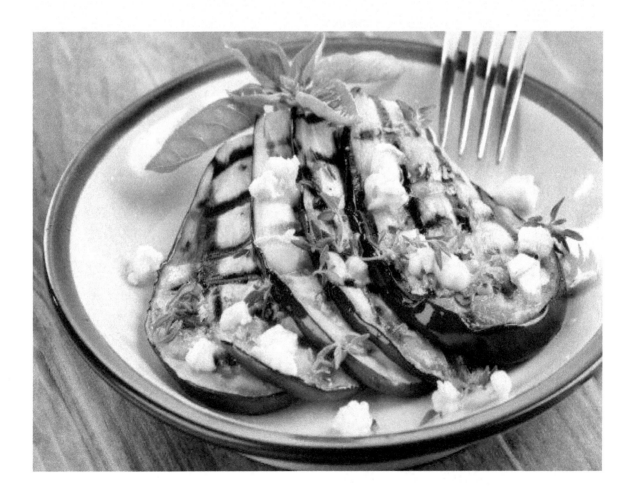

# Living the Mediterranean Way

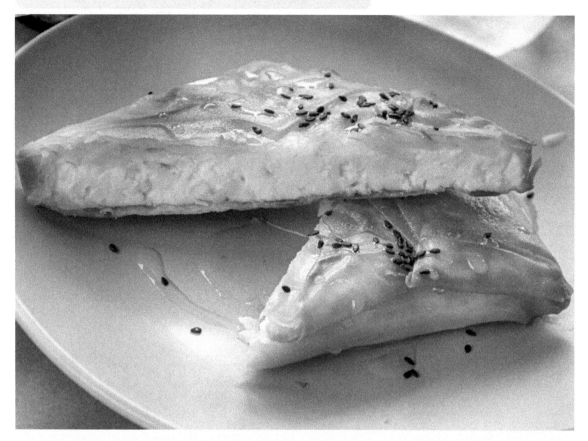

The Mediterranean region also has certain lifestyle aspects that will make a huge difference in how this diet works for you.

The Mediterranean region is, as a whole, more active. Their outdoor spaces are open and inviting (how could you not want to walk on the Mediterranean beach), and they have shorter commute times that usually render a car unnecessary. These mild things make a difference, and with these changes, they naturally make time for exercise too.

These changes can affect your metabolism and make a huge difference in how your body might handle things! You can try to go out for morning walks, or find some workout videos if you have an area at home. Going to a gym regularly can also be of great benefit.

The Mediterranean region is also in the habit of being social when it comes to food. Eating with the family, and having big gatherings that surround food as a culture are major. They also take time with lunch, even on the working day. Eating with people encourages you to slow down and taste what you are eating. You won't be trying to get it all down as quickly as possible.

Finally, they are wary of processed and outsourced food items. They can get everything they need rather easily, so why would they need anything processed. Processed and outsourced items can cost more in this region.

Small changes like these make a world of difference. The data proves it!

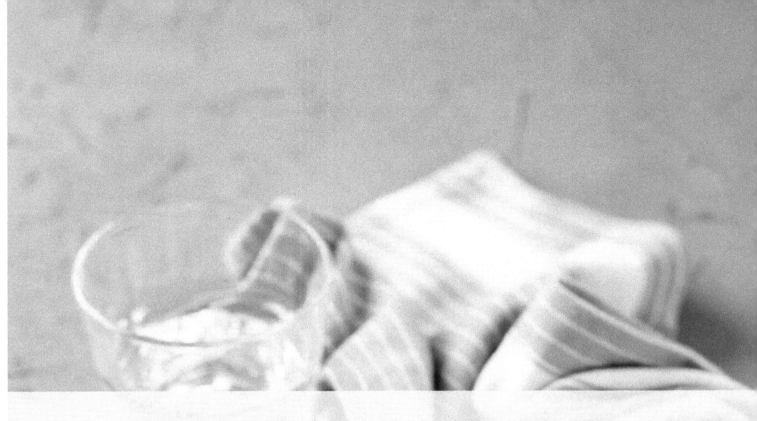

# CHAPTER 3: BEANS AND GRAINS

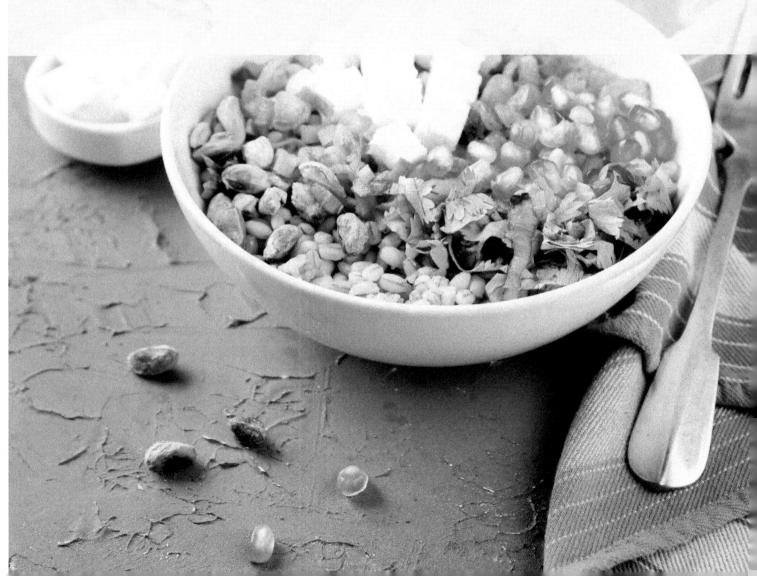

# Chapter 3: Beans And Grains

## Barley Salad with Lemon-Tahini Dressing

**Prep time: 15 minutes | Cook time: 10 minutes | Serves 4 to 6**
1½ cups (187 g) pearl barley
5 tablespoons (75 ml) extra-virgin olive oil, divided
1½ teaspoons (6 g) table salt, for cooking barley
¼ cup (60 g) tahini
1 teaspoon(5 g) grated lemon zest plus ¼ cup (60 ml) juice (2 lemons)
1 tablespoon(15 g) sumac, divided
1 garlic clove, minced
¾ teaspoon(4 g) table salt
1 English cucumber, cut into ½-inch pieces
1 carrot, peeled and shredded
1 red bell pepper, stemmed, seeded, and chopped
4 scallions, sliced thin
2 tablespoons (30 g) finely chopped jarred hot cherry peppers
¼ (5 g)cup coarsely chopped fresh mint

1. Combine 6 cups water, barley, 1 tablespoon oil, and 1½ teaspoons salt in Instant Pot. Lock lid in place and close pressure release valve. Select high pressure cook function and cook for 8 minutes. Turn off Instant Pot and let pressure release naturally for 15 minutes. Quick-release any remaining pressure, then carefully remove lid, allowing steam to escape away from you. Drain barley, spread onto rimmed baking sheet, and let cool completely, about 15 minutes. 2. Meanwhile, whisk remaining ¼ cup oil, tahini, 2 tablespoons water, lemon zest and juice, 1 teaspoon sumac, garlic, and ¾ teaspoon salt in large bowl until combined; let sit for 15 minutes. 3. Measure out and reserve ½ cup dressing for serving. Add barley, cucumber, carrot, bell pepper, scallions, and cherry peppers to bowl with dressing and gently toss to combine. Season with salt and pepper to taste. Transfer salad to serving dish and sprinkle with mint and remaining 2 teaspoons sumac. Serve, passing reserved dressing separately.
**Per Serving**
Calories: 370 | fat: 18g | protein: 8g | carbs: 47g | fiber: 10g | sodium: 510mg

# Lentil Chili

**Prep time: 15 minutes | Cook time: 30 minutes | Serves 6**
2 tablespoons (30 ml) olive oil
1 medium yellow onion, peeled and chopped
1 large poblano pepper, seeded and chopped
¼ cup (5 g)chopped fresh cilantro
2 cloves garlic, peeled and minced
1 tablespoon (15 g) chili powder
½ teaspoon (3 g) ground cumin
½ teaspoon (3 g) ground black pepper
¼ teaspoon (1 g)salt
2 cups (250 g) dried red lentils, rinsed and drained
6 cups (1500 ml) vegetable broth
1 (10-ounce / 283-g) can tomatoes with green chilies, drained
1 (15-ounce / 425-g) can kidney beans, drained and rinsed
1 tablespoon (15 ml) lime juice

1. Press the Sauté button on the Instant Pot® and heat oil. Add onion and poblano pepper, and cook until just tender, about 3 minutes. Add cilantro, garlic, chili powder, cumin, black pepper, and salt, and cook until fragrant, about 30 seconds. Press the Cancel button. 2. Add lentils and broth, close lid, set steam release to Sealing, press the Manual button, and set time to 25 minutes. When the timer beeps, let pressure release naturally, about 15 minutes. 3. Open lid and stir in tomatoes, beans, and lime juice. Let stand uncovered on the Keep Warm setting for 10 minutes. Serve warm.

**Per Serving**
Calories: 261 | fat: 6g | protein: 15g | carbs: 42g | fiber: 9g | sodium: 781mg

# Greek-Style Lentils

**Prep time: 10 minutes | Cook time: 6 minutes | Serves 6**
1 cup (125 g) dried black lentils, rinsed and drained
2 cups (500 ml)water
½ medium red onion, peeled and diced
¼ cup (31 g) chopped sun-dried tomatoes
¼ cup (31 g)chopped Kalamata olives
2 tablespoons (30 g) chopped fresh basil
2 tablespoons (30 g) chopped fresh Italian parsley
¼ cup (63 ml) extra-virgin olive oil
¼ cup (63 ml) lemon juice
2 tablespoons (30 ml) red wine vinegar
1 tablespoon (18 g) tahini

1 clove garlic, peeled and minced

¼ teaspoon (1 g) salt

¼ teaspoon (1 g) ground black pepper

1. Add lentils and water to the Instant Pot®. Close lid, set steam release to Sealing, press the Manual button, and set time to 6 minutes. When the timer beeps, let pressure release naturally for 15 minutes, then quick-release any remaining pressure until the float valve drops. Open lid and drain off any excess liquid. 2. Transfer lentils to a large bowl. Stir in onion, sun-dried tomatoes, olives, basil, and parsley. In a small bowl, combine oil, lemon juice, vinegar, tahini, garlic, salt, and pepper, and whisk to mix. Pour dressing over lentil mixture and toss to coat. Serve warm or at room temperature.

**Per Serving**

Calories: 200 | fat: 14g | protein: 5g | carbs: 15g | fiber: 2g | sodium: 250mg

# Cilantro Lime Rice

**Prep time: 10 minutes | Cook time: 32 minutes | Serves 8**

2 tablespoons (30 ml) extra-virgin olive oil

½ medium yellow onion, peeled and chopped

2 cloves garlic, peeled and minced

½ cup (10 g) chopped fresh cilantro, divided

2 cups (250 g) brown rice

2¼ cups (563 ml) water

2 tablespoons (30 ml) lime juice

1 tablespoon (15 g) grated lime zest

¼ teaspoon (1 g) salt

½ teaspoon (3 g) ground black pepper

1. Press the Sauté button on the Instant Pot® and heat oil. Add onion and cook until soft, about 6 minutes. Add garlic and ¼ cup cilantro and cook until fragrant, about 30 seconds. Add rice and cook, stirring constantly, until well coated and starting to toast, about 3 minutes. Press the Cancel button. 2. Stir in water. Close lid, set steam release to Sealing, press the Manual button, and set time to 22 minutes. When the timer beeps, let pressure release naturally for 10 minutes, then quick-release the remaining pressure. Open lid and fluff rice with a fork. Fold in remaining ¼ cup cilantro, lime juice, lime zest, salt, and pepper. Serve warm.

**Per Serving**

Calories: 95 | fat: 4g | protein: 1g | carbs: 14g | fiber: 1g | sodium: 94mg

# Mediterranean Creamed Green Peas

**Prep time: 5 minutes | Cook time: 25 minutes | Serves 4**
1 cup (125 g) cauliflower florets, fresh or frozen
½ white onion, roughly chopped
2 tablespoons (30 ml) olive oil
½ cup (125 ml) unsweetened almond milk
3 cups (375 g) green split peas, fresh or frozen
3 garlic cloves, minced
2 tablespoons (30 g) fresh thyme leaves, chopped
1 teaspoon (1 g) fresh rosemary leaves, chopped
½ teaspoon (3 g) salt
½ teaspoon (3 g) black pepper
Shredded Parmesan cheese, for garnish
Fresh parsley, for garnish

1. Preheat the air fryer to 380°F(193°C). 2. In a large bowl, combine the cauliflower florets and onion with the olive oil and toss well to coat. 3. Put the cauliflower-and-onion mixture into the air fryer basket in an even layer and bake for 15 minutes. 4. Transfer the cauliflower and onion to a food processor. Add the almond milk and pulse until smooth. 5. In a medium saucepan, combine the cauliflower purée, peas, garlic, thyme, rosemary, salt, and pepper and mix well. Cook over medium heat for an additional 10 minutes, stirring regularly. 6. Serve with a sprinkle of Parmesan cheese and chopped fresh parsley.
**Per Serving**
Calories: 313 | fat: 16.4g | protein: 14.7g | carbs: 28.8g | fiber: 8.3g | sodium: 898mg

# Moroccan Date Pilaf

**Prep time: 10 minutes | Cook time: 30 minutes | Serves 4**
3 tablespoons (45 ml) olive oil
1 onion, chopped
3 garlic cloves, minced
1 cup (125 g) uncooked long-grain rice
½ to 1 tablespoon (7.5-15 g) harissa
5 or 6 Medjool dates (or another variety), pitted and chopped
¼ cup (31 g) dried cranberries
¼ teaspoon (1 g) ground cinnamon
½ teaspoon (3 g) ground turmeric
¼ teaspoon (1 g) sea salt
¼ teaspoon (1 g) freshly ground black pepper

2 cups (500 ml) chicken broth
¼ cup (31 g) shelled whole pistachios, for garnish

1. In a large stockpot, heat the olive oil over medium heat. Add the onion and garlic and sauté for 3 to 5 minutes, until the onion is soft. Add the rice and cook for 3 minutes, until the grains start to turn opaque. Add the harissa, dates, cranberries, cinnamon, turmeric, salt, and pepper and cook for 30 seconds. Add the broth and bring to a boil, then reduce the heat to low, cover, and simmer for 20 minutes, or until the liquid has been absorbed. 2. Remove the rice from the heat and stir in the nuts. Let stand for 10 minutes before serving.

**Per Serving**
Calories: 368 | fat: 15g | protein: 6g | carbs: 54g | fiber: 4g | sodium: 83mg

# Vegetable Barley Soup

**Prep time: 30 minutes | Cook time: 26 minutes | Serves 8**
2 tablespoons (30 ml) olive oil
½ medium yellow onion, peeled and chopped
1 medium carrot, peeled and chopped
1 stalk celery, chopped
2 cups (250 g) sliced button mushrooms
2 cloves garlic, peeled and minced
½ teaspoon (3 g) dried thyme
½ teaspoon (3 g) ground black pepper
1 large russet potato, peeled and cut into ½" pieces
1(14½-ounce / 411-g) can fire-roasted diced tomatoes, undrained
½ cup (63 g) medium pearl barley, rinsed and drained
4 cups (1000 ml) vegetable broth
2 cups (500 ml) water
1 (15-ounce / 425-g) can corn, drained
1 (15-ounce / 425-g) can cut green beans, drained
1 (15-ounce / 425-g) can Great Northern beans, drained and rinsed
½ teaspoon (3 g) salt

1. Press the Sauté button on the Instant Pot® and heat oil. Add onion, carrot, celery, and mushrooms. Cook until just tender, about 5 minutes. Add garlic, thyme, and pepper. Cook 30 seconds. Press the Cancel button. 2. Add potato, tomatoes, barley, broth, and water to pot. Close lid, set steam release to Sealing, press the Soup button, and cook for the default time of 20 minutes. 3. When the timer beeps, let pressure release naturally, about 15 minutes. Open lid and stir soup, then add corn, green beans, and Great Northern beans. Close lid and let stand on the Keep Warm setting for 10 minutes. Stir in salt. Serve hot.

**Per Serving**

Calories: 190 | fat: 4g | protein: 7g | carbs: 34g | fiber: 8g | sodium: 548mg

# White Bean and Barley Soup

**Prep time: 20 minutes | Cook time: 26 minutes | Serves 8**

2 tablespoons (30 ml) light olive oil

½ medium onion, peeled and chopped

1 medium carrot, peeled and chopped

1 stalk celery, chopped

2 cloves garlic, peeled and minced

2 sprigs fresh thyme

1 bay leaf

½ teaspoon (3 g) ground black pepper

1 (14-ounce / 397-g) can fire-roasted diced tomatoes, undrained

½ cup (63 g) medium pearl barley, rinsed and drained

4 cups (1000 ml) vegetable broth

2 cups (500 ml) water

2 (15-ounce / 425-g) cans Great Northern beans, drained and rinsed

½ teaspoon (3 g) salt

1. Press the Sauté button on the Instant Pot® and heat oil. Add onion, carrot, and celery. Cook until just tender, about 5 minutes. Add garlic, thyme, bay leaf, and pepper, and cook until fragrant, about 30 seconds. Press the Cancel button. 2. Add the tomatoes, barley, broth, and water. Close lid, set steam release to Sealing, press the Soup button, and cook for default time of 20 minutes. 3. When the timer beeps, let pressure release naturally, about 20 minutes. Open lid, stir soup, then add beans and salt. Close lid and let stand on the Keep Warm setting for 10 minutes. Remove and discard bay leaf. Serve hot.

**Per Serving**

Calories: 129 | fat: 4g | protein: 5g | carbs: 20g | fiber: 5g | sodium: 636mg

# Chickpeas with Spinach and Sun-Dried Tomatoes

**Prep time: 10 minutes | Cook time: 2 hours 30 minutes | Serves 3**
½ pound (227 g) uncooked chickpeas
4 tablespoons (60 ml) extra virgin olive oil, divided
2 spring onions (white parts only), sliced
1 small onion (any variety), diced
1 pound (454 g) fresh spinach, washed and chopped
½ cup (125 ml) white wine
½ cup (63 g) sun-dried tomatoes (packed in oil), drained, rinsed, and chopped
1 tablespoon (15 g) chopped fresh mint
1 tablespoon (15 g) chopped fresh dill
6 tablespoons (90 ml) fresh lemon juice, divided
¼ teaspoon (1 g) freshly ground black pepper
¾ (1 g) teaspoon fine sea salt

1. Place the chickpeas in a large bowl and cover with cold water by 3 inches (7.5cm) to allow for expansion. Soak overnight or for 12 hours. 2. When ready to cook, drain and rinse the chickpeas. Place them in a large pot and cover with cold water. Place the pot over high heat and bring to a boil (using a slotted spoon to remove any foam), then reduce the heat to low and simmer until the chickpeas are tender but not falling apart, about 1 to 1½ hours, checking the chickpeas every 30 minutes to ensure they aren't overcooking. Use the slotted spoon to transfer the chickpeas a medium bowl and then reserve the cooking water. Set aside. 3. In a deep pan, heat 3 tablespoons of the olive oil over medium heat. When the oil begins to shimmer, add the spring onions and diced onions, and sauté for 5 minutes or until soft, then add the spinach. Toss and continue cooking for 5–7 minutes or until the spinach has wilted. Add the wine and continue cooking for 2 minutes or until the liquid has evaporated. 4. Add the cooked chickpeas, sun-dried tomatoes, mint, dill, 3 tablespoons of the lemon juice, black pepper, and 1½ cups of the chickpea cooking water. Bring the mixture to a boil and then reduce the heat to low and simmer for 30–45 minutes or until the liquid has been absorbed and the chickpeas have thickened, adding more water as needed if the chickpeas appear to be too dry. About 5 minutes before removing the chickpeas from the heat, add the remaining 1 tablespoon of olive oil, a tablespoon of the lemon juice, and the sea salt. Mix well, then remove the pan from the heat, keeping it covered, and set aside to rest for 5 minutes. 5. Divide the mixture between three bowls and top each serving with 1 tablespoon of the lemon juice. Store covered in the refrigerator for up to 3 days.
**Per Serving**
Calories: 599 | fat: 24g | protein: 24g | carbs: 81g | fiber: 17g | sodium: 764mg

# Orzo-Veggie Pilaf

**Prep time: 20 minutes | Cook time: 10 minutes | Serves 6**
2 cups (250 g) orzo
1 pint (2 cups / 250-g) cherry tomatoes, cut in half
1 cup (125 g) Kalamata olives
½ cup (10 g) fresh basil, finely chopped
½ cup (125 ml) extra-virgin olive oil

⅓ cup balsamic vinegar

1 teaspoon (5 g) salt
½ teaspoon (3 g) freshly ground black pepper

1. Bring a large pot of water to a boil. Add the orzo and cook for 7 minutes.
Drain and rinse the orzo with cold water in a strainer. 2. Once the orzo has
cooled, put it in a large bowl. Add the tomatoes, olives, and basil. 3. In a small
bowl, whisk together the olive oil, vinegar, salt, and pepper. Add this dressing
to the pasta and toss everything together. Serve at room temperature or
chilled.

**Per Serving**
Calories: 476 | fat: 28g | protein: 8g | carbs: 48g | fiber: 3g | sodium: 851mg

# Sea Salt Soybeans

**Prep time: 5 minutes | Cook time: 12 minutes | Serves 4**
1 cup (125 g) shelled edamame
8 cups (2000 ml) water, divided
1 tablespoon (15 ml) vegetable oil
1 teaspoon (5 g) coarse sea salt
2 tablespoons (30 ml) soy sauce

1. Add edamame and 4 cups water to the Instant Pot®. Close lid, set steam
release to Sealing, and set time to 1 minute. When the timer beeps,
quick-release the pressure until the float valve drops. Press the Cancel button.
2. Open lid, drain and rinse edamame, and return to pot with the remaining 4
cups water. Soak for 1 hour. 3. Add oil. Close lid, set steam release to Sealing,
press the Manual button, and set time to 11 minutes. When the timer beeps,
let pressure release naturally, about 25 minutes, then open lid. 4. Drain
edamame and transfer to a serving bowl. Sprinkle with salt and serve with soy
sauce on the side for dipping.

**Per Serving**
Calories: 76 | fat: 5g | protein: 4g | carbs: 5g | fiber: 2g | sodium: 768mg

# Moroccan White Beans with Lamb

**Prep time: 25 minutes | Cook time: 22 minutes | Serves 6 to 8**

1½ tablespoons (22 g) table salt, for brining

1 pound (454 g) dried great Northern beans, picked over and rinsed

1 (12-ounce/ 340-g) lamb shoulder chop (blade or round bone), ¾ to 1 inch thick, trimmed and halved

½ teaspoon (3 g) table salt

2 tablespoons (30 ml) extra-virgin olive oil, plus extra for serving

1 onion, chopped

1 red bell pepper, stemmed, seeded, and chopped

2 tablespoons (36 g) tomato paste

3 garlic cloves, minced

2 teaspoons (10 g) paprika

2 teaspoons (10 g) ground cumin

1½ teaspoon (3 g)s ground ginger

¼ teaspoon (1 g) cayenne pepper

½ cup (125 ml) dry white wine

2 cups (500 ml) chicken broth

2 tablespoons (30 g) minced fresh parsley

1. Dissolve 1½ tablespoons salt in 2 quarts cold water in large container. Add beans and soak at room temperature for at least 8 hours or up to 24 hours. Drain and rinse well. 2. Pat lamb dry with paper towels and sprinkle with ½ teaspoon salt. Using highest sauté function, heat oil in Instant Pot for 5 minutes (or until just smoking). Brown lamb, about 5 minutes per side; transfer to plate. 3. Add onion and bell pepper to fat left in pot and cook, using highest sauté function, until softened, about 5 minutes. Stir in tomato paste, garlic, paprika, cumin, ginger, and cayenne and cook until fragrant, about 30 seconds. Stir in wine, scraping up any browned bits, then stir in broth and beans. 4. Nestle lamb into beans and add any accumulated juices. Lock lid in place and close pressure release valve. Select high pressure cook function and cook for 1 minute. Turn off Instant Pot and let pressure release naturally for 15 minutes. Quick-release any remaining pressure, then carefully remove lid, allowing steam to escape away from you. 5. Transfer lamb to cutting board, let cool slightly, then shred into bite-size pieces using 2 forks; discard excess fat and bones. Stir lamb and parsley into beans, and season with salt and pepper to taste. Drizzle individual portions with extra oil before serving.

**Per Serving**

Calories: 350 | fat: 12g | protein: 20g | carbs: 40g | fiber: 15g | sodium: 410mg

# Earthy Lentil and Rice Pilaf

**Prep time: 5 minutes | Cook time: 50 minutes | Serves 6**

¼ cup (63 ml) extra-virgin olive oil

1 large onion, chopped

6 cups (1500 ml) water

1 teaspoon (5 g) ground cumin

1 teaspoon (5 g) salt

2 cups (250 g) brown lentils, picked over and rinsed

1 cup (125 g) basmati rice

1. In a medium pot over medium heat, cook the olive oil and onions for 7 to 10 minutes until the edges are browned. 2. Turn the heat to high, add the water, cumin, and salt, and bring this mixture to a boil, boiling for about 3 minutes. 3. Add the lentils and turn the heat to medium-low. Cover the pot and cook for 20 minutes, stirring occasionally. 4. Stir in the rice and cover; cook for an additional 20 minutes. 5. Fluff the rice with a fork and serve warm.

**Per Serving**

Calories: 397 | fat: 11g | protein: 18g | carbs: 60g | fiber: 18g | sodium: 396mg

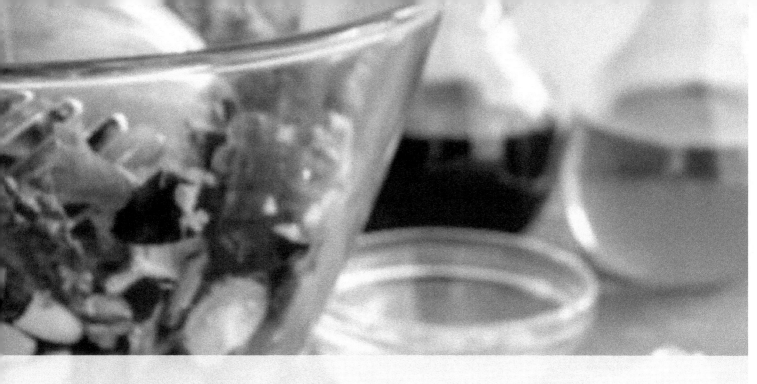

# CHAPTER 4: VEGETABLES AND SIDES

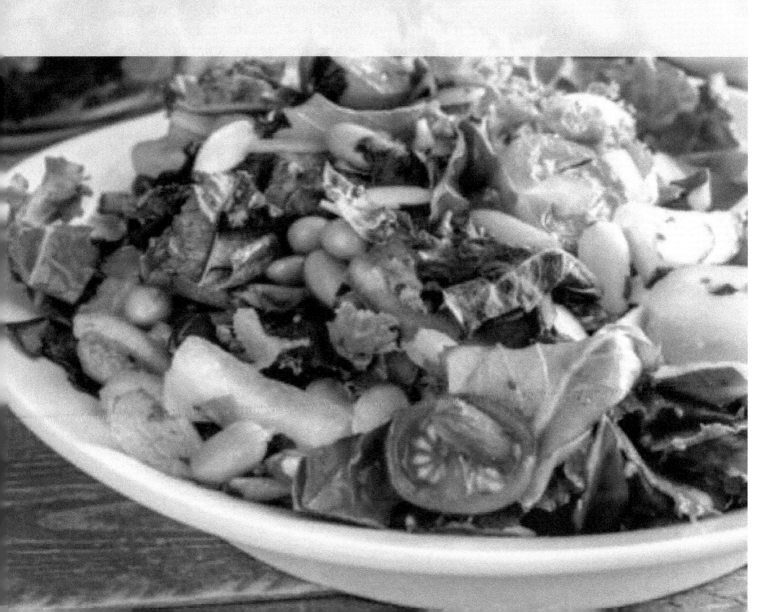

# Chapter 4: Vegetables And Sides

## Individual Asparagus and Goat Cheese Frittatas

**Prep time: 15 minutes | Cook time: 15 minutes | Serves 4**
1 tablespoon (15 ml) extra-virgin olive oil
8 ounces (227 g) asparagus, trimmed and sliced ¼ inch thick
1 red bell pepper, stemmed, seeded, and chopped
2 shallots, minced
2 ounces (57 g) goat cheese, crumbled (½ cup)
1 tablespoon (15 g) minced fresh tarragon
1 teaspoon (1 g) grated lemon zest
8 large eggs
½ teaspoon (3 g) table salt

1. Using highest sauté function, heat oil in Instant Pot until shimmering. Add asparagus, bell pepper, and shallots; cook until softened, about 5 minutes. Turn off Instant Pot and transfer vegetables to bowl. Stir in goat cheese, tarragon, and lemon zest. 2. Arrange trivet included with Instant Pot in base of now-empty insert and add 1 cup water. Spray four 6-ounce ramekins with vegetable oil spray. Beat eggs, ¼ cup water, and salt in large bowl until thoroughly combined. Divide vegetable mixture between prepared ramekins, then pour egg mixture over top (you may have some left over). Set ramekins on trivet. Lock lid in place and close pressure release valve. Select high pressure cook function and cook for 10 minutes. 3. Turn off Instant Pot and quick-release pressure. Carefully remove lid, allowing steam to escape away from you. Using tongs, transfer ramekins to wire rack and let cool slightly. Run paring knife around inside edge of ramekins to loosen frittatas, then invert onto individual serving plates. Serve.

**Per Serving**
Calories: 240 | fat: 16g | protein: 17g | carbs: 6g | fiber: 2g | sodium: 500mg

# Vegetable Tagine

**Prep time: 15 minutes | Cook time: 45 minutes | Serves 4**
3 tablespoons (45 ml) olive oil
1 onion, thinly sliced
5 garlic cloves, minced
2 carrots, cut into long ribbons
2 red bell peppers, coarsely chopped
1 (15-ounce / 425-g) can diced tomatoes
½ cup (63 g) chopped dried apricots
1 to 2 tablespoons (18-36 g) harissa
1 teaspoon (1 g) ground coriander
½ teaspoon (3 g) ground turmeric
½ teaspoon (3 g) ground cinnamon
3 cups (750 ml) vegetable broth
1 sweet potato, peeled and cubed
1 (15-ounce / 425-g) can chickpeas, drained and rinsed
Sea salt
Freshly ground black pepper

1. In a large stockpot, heat the olive oil over medium-high heat. Add the onion and garlic and sauté for 5 minutes. Add the carrots and bell peppers and sauté for 7 to 10 minutes, until the vegetables are tender. 2. Add the tomatoes, apricots, harissa, coriander, turmeric, and cinnamon and cook for 5 minutes. Add the broth and sweet potato and bring to a boil. Reduce the heat to low, cover, and simmer for 20 minutes, or until the sweet potato is tender. 3. Add the chickpeas and simmer for 3 minutes to heat through. Season with salt and black pepper and serve.

**Per Serving**
Calories: 324 | fat: 12g | protein: 9g | carbs: 48g | fiber: 12g | sodium: 210mg

# Lightened-Up Eggplant Parmigiana

**Prep time: 10 minutes | Cook time: 1 hour 20 minutes | Serves 3**
2 medium globe eggplants, sliced into ¼-inch rounds
2 tablespoons (30 ml) extra virgin olive oil, divided
1 teaspoon (5 g) fine sea salt, divided
1 medium onion (any variety), diced
1 garlic clove, finely chopped
20 ounces (567g) canned crushed tomatoes or tomato purée
3 tablespoons (3 g) chopped fresh basil, divided
¼ teaspoon (1 g) freshly ground black pepper
7 ounces (198 g) low-moisture mozzarella, thinly sliced or grated

2 ounces (57 g) grated Parmesan cheese

1. Line an oven rack with aluminum foil and preheat the oven to 350°F (180°C). 2. Place the eggplant slices in a large bowl and toss with 1 tablespoon of the olive oil and ½ teaspoon of the sea salt. Arrange the slices on the prepared oven rack. Place the oven rack in the middle position and roast the eggplant for 15–20 minutes or until soft. 3. While the eggplant slices are roasting, heat the remaining tablespoon of olive oil in a medium pan over medium heat. When the oil begins to shimmer, add the onions and sauté for 5 minutes, then add the garlic and sauté for 1 more minute. Add the crushed tomatoes, 1½ tablespoons of the basil, the remaining ½ teaspoon of sea salt, and black pepper. Reduce the heat to low and simmer for 15 minutes, then remove from the heat. 4. When the eggplant slices are done roasting, remove them from the oven. Begin assembling the dish by spreading ½ cup of the tomato sauce over the bottom of a 11 × 7-inch (30 × 20cm) casserole dish. Place a third of the eggplant rounds in a single layer in the dish, overlapping them slightly, if needed. Layer half of the mozzarella on top of the eggplant, then spread ¾ cup tomato sauce over the cheese slices and then sprinkle 2½ tablespoons of the grated Parmesan cheese over the top. Repeat the process with a second layer of eggplant, sauce, and cheese, then add the remaining eggplant in a single layer on top of the cheese. Top with the remaining sauce and then sprinkle the remaining 1½ tablespoons of basil over the top. 5. Bake for 40–45 minutes or until browned, then remove from oven and set aside to cool for 10 minutes before cutting into 6 equal-size pieces and serving. Store covered in the refrigerator for up to 3 days.

**Per Serving**
Calories: 453 | fat: 28g | protein: 28g | carbs: 26g | fiber: 4g | sodium: 842mg

# Rice Pilaf with Dill

**Prep time: 15 minutes | Cook time: 25 minutes | Serves 6**
2 tablespoons (30 ml) olive oil
1 carrot, finely chopped (about ¾ cup)
2 leeks, halved lengthwise, washed, well drained, and sliced in half-moons
½ teaspoon (3 g) salt
¼ teaspoon (1 g) freshly ground black pepper
2 tablespoons (30 g) chopped fresh dill
1 cup (250 ml) low-sodium vegetable broth or water
½ cup (63 g) basmati rice

1. In a 2-or 3-quart saucepan, heat the olive oil over medium heat. Add the carrot, leeks, salt, pepper, and 1 tablespoon of the dill. Cover and cook for 6 to 8 minutes, stirring once, to soften all the vegetables but not brown them. 2. Add the broth or water and bring to a boil. Stir in the rice, reduce the heat to

maintain a simmer, cover, and cook for 15 minutes. Remove from the heat; let stand, covered, for 10 minutes. 3. Fluff the rice with fork. Stir in the remaining 1 tablespoon dill and serve.

**Per Serving**1 cup:

Calories: 100 | fat: 7g | protein: 2g | carbs: 11g | fiber: 4g | sodium: 209mg

# Lemon-Rosemary Beets

**Prep time: 10 minutes | Cook time: 8 hours | Serves 7**

2 pounds (907 g) beets, peeled and cut into wedges

2 tablespoons (30 ml) fresh lemon juice

2 tablespoons (30 ml) extra-virgin olive oil

2 tablespoons (30 ml) honey

1 tablespoon (15 ml) apple cider vinegar

¾ teaspoon sea salt

½ teaspoon (3 g) black pepper

2 sprigs fresh rosemary

½ teaspoon (3 g) lemon zest

1. Place the beets in the slow cooker. 2. Whisk the lemon juice, extra-virgin olive oil, honey, apple cider vinegar, salt, and pepper together in a small bowl. Pour over the beets. 3. Add the sprigs of rosemary to the slow cooker. 4. Cover and cook on low for 8 hours, or until the beets are tender. 5. Remove and discard the rosemary sprigs. Stir in the lemon zest. Serve hot.

**Per Serving**

Calories: 111 | fat: 4g | protein: 2g | carbs: 18g | fiber: 4g | sodium: 351mg

# Couscous-Stuffed Eggplants

**Prep time: 10 minutes | Cook time: 45 minutes | Serves 4**

2 medium eggplants (about 8 ounces / 227 g each)

1 tablespoon (15 ml) olive oil

⅓ cup whole-wheat couscous

3 tablespoons (45 g) diced dried apricots

4 scallions, thinly sliced

1 large tomato, seeded and diced

2 tablespoons (30 g) chopped fresh mint leaves

1 tablespoon (15 g) chopped, toasted pine nuts

1 tablespoon (15 ml) lemon juice

½ teaspoon (3 g) salt

¼ teaspoon (1 g) freshly ground black pepper

1. Preheat the oven to 400°F (205°C). 2. Halve the eggplants lengthwise and score the cut sides with a knife, cutting all the way through the flesh but being careful not to cut through the skin. Brush the cut sides with the olive oil and place the eggplant halves, cut-side up, on a large, rimmed baking sheet. Roast in the preheated oven for about 20 to 30 minutes, until the flesh is softened. 3. While the eggplant is roasting, place the couscous in a small saucepan or heat-safe bowl and cover with boiling water. Cover and let stand until the couscous is tender and has absorbed the water, about 10 minutes. 4. When the eggplants are soft, remove them from the oven (don't turn the oven off) and scoop the flesh into a large bowl, leaving a bit of eggplant inside the skin so that the skin holds its shape. Be cautious not to break the skin. Chop or mash the eggplant flesh and add the couscous, dried apricots, scallions, tomato, mint, pine nuts, lemon juice, salt, and pepper and stir to mix well. 5. Spoon the couscous mixture into the eggplant skins and return them to the baking sheet. Bake in the oven for another 15 minutes or so, until heated through. Serve hot.

**Per Serving**
Calories: 146 | fat: 5g | protein: 4g | carbs: 22g | fiber: 6g | sodium: 471mg

## Stuffed Eggplant with Onion and Tomato

**Prep time: 10 minutes | Cook time:1 hour 30 minutes | Serves 4**
4 medium, long eggplant, washed and stemmed
6 tablespoons (90 ml) extra virgin olive oil, divided, plus 1 teaspoon for brushing
1⅛ teaspoon fine sea salt, divided
3 medium red onions, finely chopped
5 garlic cloves, finely chopped
1 teaspoon (5 g) granulated sugar
15 ounces (425 g) chopped tomatoes (fresh or canned)
1 cinnamon stick
½ cup (30 g) chopped fresh parsley
¼ teaspoon (1 g) freshly ground black pepper
4 tablespoons (60 g) crumbled feta
4 cherry tomatoes, sliced

1. Preheat the oven to 400°F (205°C). Make 3 end-to-end slits, each about 1 inch deep, along the length of each eggplant, making sure not to cut completely through. (The slits should be about ¾ inch apart.) 2. Place the eggplant in a large baking pan, slit side up. Brush with 1 teaspoon of the olive oil, and season with ⅛ teaspoon of the sea salt. Transfer to the oven and roast for 45 minutes. 3. While the eggplant are roasting, begin preparing the filling by heating 3 tablespoons of the olive oil in a deep pan placed over medium heat. When the oil starts to shimmer, add the onions and garlic and sauté for 3

minutes. 4. Sprinkle the sugar and ¼ teaspoon of the sea salt over the onions. Stir, then reduce the heat to medium-low and cook for 15 minutes or until the onions are caramelized. (Reduce the heat if the onions begin to burn.) 5. Add the tomatoes, cinnamon stick, parsley, black pepper, and remaining ¾ teaspoon of sea salt. Stir, increase the heat to medium, and cook for 3–4 minutes. 6. When the eggplant are done roasting, remove them from the oven, carefully pull the slits open, and stuff each eggplant with the filling. 7. Place the stuffed eggplant snugly in a baking dish. Drizzle the remaining 3 tablespoons of olive oil over the eggplant, ensuring the outsides of the eggplant are coated with the oil. Sprinkle 1 tablespoon of feta over each eggplant and then top with 3–4 slices of cherry tomatoes. 8. Place the stuffed eggplant back in the oven and bake for 15 minutes, then lower the heat to 350°F (180°C) and bake for 30 more minutes. Remove from the oven and set aside to cool for at least 15 minutes before serving. Store covered in the refrigerator for up to 3 days.

**Per Serving**

Calories: 408 | fat: 24g | protein: 9g | carbs: 48g | fiber: 20g | sodium: 771mg

# Egg Casserole with Tomato, Spinach, and Feta

**Prep time: 10 minutes | Cook time: 6 to 8 hours | Serves 6**

12 large eggs
¼ cup (63 ml) milk of your choice
1 cup (125 g) fresh spinach, chopped
¼ cup (63 g) feta cheese, crumbled
½ teaspoon (3 g) sea salt
¼ teaspoon (1 g) freshly ground black pepper
Nonstick cooking spray
2 Roma tomatoes, sliced

1. In a medium bowl, whisk together the eggs, milk, spinach, feta cheese, salt, and pepper until combined. 2. Generously coat a slow-cooker insert with cooking spray. 3. Pour the egg mixture into the slow cooker. Top with the tomato slices. 4. Cover the cooker and cook for 6 to 8 hours on Low heat.

**Per Serving**

Calories: 178 | fat: 11g | protein: 14g | carbs: 4g | fiber: 1g | sodium: 416mg

# Moroccan-Style Couscous

**Prep time: 10 minutes | Cook time: 5 minutes | Serves 2**
1 tablespoon (15 ml) olive oil
¾ cup (1 g) couscous
¼ teaspoon (1 g) garlic powder
¼ teaspoon (1 g) salt
¼ teaspoon (1 g) cinnamon
1 cup (250 ml) water
2 tablespoons (30 g) raisins
2 tablespoons (30 g) minced dried apricots
2 teaspoons (2 g) minced fresh parsley

1. Heat the olive oil in a saucepan over medium-high heat. Add the couscous, garlic powder, salt, and cinnamon. Stir for 1 minute to toast the couscous and spices. 2. Add the water, raisins, and apricots and bring the mixture to a boil. 3. Cover the pot and turn off the heat. Let the couscous sit for 4 to 5 minutes and then fluff it with a fork. Add parsley and season with additional salt or spices as needed.

**Per Serving**
Calories: 338 | fat: 8g | protein: 9g | carbs: 59g | fiber: 4g | sodium: 299mg

# Roasted Broccoli with Tahini Yogurt Sauce

**Prep time: 15 minutes | Cook time: 30 minutes | Serves 4**
**For the Broccoli:**
1½ to 2 pounds (680 to 907 g) broccoli, stalk trimmed and cut into slices, head cut into florets
1 lemon, sliced into ¼-inch-thick rounds
3 tablespoons (45 ml) extra-virgin olive oil
½ teaspoon (3 g) kosher salt
¼ teaspoon (1 g) freshly ground black pepper
**For the Tahini Yogurt Sauce:**
½ cup (125 g) plain Greek yogurt
2 tablespoons (36 g) tahini
1 tablespoon (15 ml) lemon juice
¼ teaspoon (1 g) kosher salt
1 teaspoon (5 g) sesame seeds, for garnish (optional)

**Make the Broccoli:** 1. Preheat the oven to 425°F (220°C). Line a baking sheet with parchment paper or foil. 2. In a large bowl, gently toss the broccoli, lemon slices, olive oil, salt, and black pepper to combine. Arrange the broccoli in a single layer on the prepared baking sheet. Roast 15 minutes, stir, and roast another 15 minutes, until golden brown. **Make the Tahini Yogurt Sauce:** 3. In a medium bowl, combine the yogurt, tahini, lemon juice, and salt; mix well. 4. Spread the tahini yogurt sauce on a platter or large plate and top with the broccoli and lemon slices. Garnish with the sesame seeds (if desired).

**Per Serving**

Calories: 245 | fat: 16g | protein: 12g | carbs: 20g | fiber: 7g | sodium: 305mg

# Vibrant Green Beans

**Prep time: 10 minutes | Cook time: 15 minutes | Serves 6**

2 tablespoons (30 ml) olive oil

2 leeks, white parts only, sliced

Sea salt and freshly ground pepper, to taste

1 pound (454 g) fresh green string beans, trimmed

1 tablespoon (15 g) Italian seasoning

2 tablespoons (30 ml) white wine

Zest of 1 lemon

1. Heat the olive oil over medium heat in a large skillet. 2. Add leeks and cook, stirring often, until they start to brown and become lightly caramelized. 3. Season with sea salt and freshly ground pepper. 4. Add green beans and Italian seasoning, cooking for a few minutes until beans are tender but still crisp to the bite. 5. Add the wine and continue cooking until beans are done to your liking and leeks are crispy and browned. 6. Sprinkle with lemon zest before serving.

**Per Serving**

Calories: 87 | fat: 5g | protein: 2g | carbs: 11g | fiber: 3g | sodium: 114mg

# Garlicky Broccoli Rabe with Artichokes

**Prep time: 5 minutes | Cook time: 10 minutes | Serves 4**
2 pounds (907 g) fresh broccoli rabe
½ cup (125 ml) extra-virgin olive oil, divided
3 garlic cloves, finely minced
1 teaspoon (5 g) salt
1 teaspoon (1 g) red pepper flakes
1 (13¾-ounce / 390-g) can artichoke hearts, drained and quartered
1 tablespoon (15 ml) water
2 tablespoons (30 ml) red wine vinegar
Freshly ground black pepper

1. Trim away any thick lower stems and yellow leaves from the broccoli rabe and discard. Cut into individual florets with a couple inches of thin stem attached. 2. In a large skillet, heat ¼ cup olive oil over medium-high heat. Add the trimmed broccoli, garlic, salt, and red pepper flakes and sauté for 5 minutes, until the broccoli begins to soften. Add the artichoke hearts and sauté for another 2 minutes. 3. Add the water and reduce the heat to low. Cover and simmer until the broccoli stems are tender, 3 to 5 minutes. 4. In a small bowl, whisk together remaining ¼ cup olive oil and the vinegar. Drizzle over the broccoli and artichokes. Season with ground black pepper, if desired.

**Per Serving**
Calories: 341 | fat: 28g | protein: 11g | carbs: 18g | fiber: 12g | sodium: 750mg

# Savory Butternut Squash and Apples

**Prep time: 20 minutes | Cook time: 4 hours | Serves 10**
1 (3-pound / 1.4-kg) butternut squash, peeled, seeded, and cubed
4 cooking apples (granny smith or honeycrisp work well), peeled, cored, and chopped
¾ cup dried currants
½ sweet yellow onion such as vidalia, sliced thin
1 tablespoon (15 g) ground cinnamon
1½ teaspoons (7.5 g) ground nutmeg

1. Combine the squash, apples, currants, and onion in the slow cooker. Sprinkle with the cinnamon and nutmeg. 2. Cook on high for 4 hours, or until the squash is tender and cooked through. Stir occasionally while cooking.

**Per Serving**
Calories: 114 | fat: 0g | protein: 2g | carbs: 28g | fiber: 6g | sodium: 8mg

# Cretan Roasted Zucchini

**Prep time: 15 minutes | Cook time: 1 hour 15 minutes | Serves 2**
6 small zucchini (no longer than 6 inches), washed and ends trimmed
3 garlic cloves, thinly sliced
2 medium tomatoes, chopped, or 1 (15-ounce / 425-g) can crushed tomatoes

⅓ cup extra virgin olive oil

½ teaspoon (3 g) salt
½ teaspoon (3 g) freshly ground black pepper
2 tablespoons (30 g) chopped fresh parsley, divided
Coarse sea salt, for serving (optional)

1. Preheat the oven to 350°F (180°C). 2. Make a long, lengthwise slit in each zucchini that reaches about halfway through. (Do not cut the zucchini all the way through.) Stuff each zucchini with the sliced garlic. 3. Transfer the tomatoes to an oven-safe casserole dish, and nestle the zucchini between the tomatoes. Drizzle the olive oil over the zucchini and tomatoes. 4. Sprinkle the salt, black pepper, and 1 tablespoon of the parsley over the zucchini and tomatoes. Turn the zucchini gently so they are covered in the olive oil. 5. Transfer to the oven and cook for 1 hour 15 minutes or until the skins are soft and the edges have browned. 6. Carefully remove the dish from the oven and sprinkle the remaining parsley and sea salt, if using, over the top. Store covered in the refrigerator for up to 3 days.

**Per Serving**
Calories: 406 | fat: 37g | protein: 6g | carbs: 18g | fiber: 5g | sodium: 619mg

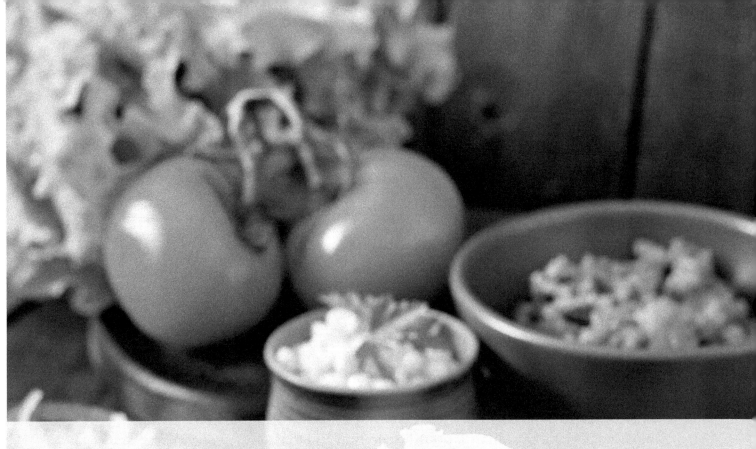

# CHAPTER 5: BREAKFAST

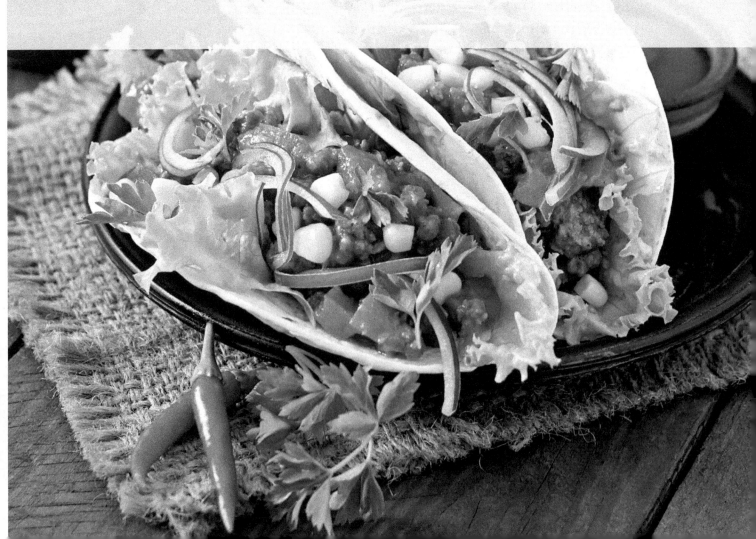

# Chapter 5: Breakfast

## Jalapeño Popper Egg Cups

**Prep time: 10 minutes | Cook time: 10 minutes | Serves 2**
4 large eggs
¼ cup (31 g) chopped pickled jalapeños
2 ounces (57 g) full-fat cream cheese
½ cup (125 g) shredded sharp Cheddar cheese

1. In a medium bowl, beat the eggs, then pour into four silicone muffin cups. 2. In a large microwave-safe bowl, place jalapeños, cream cheese, and Cheddar. Microwave for 30 seconds and stir. Take a spoonful, approximately ¼ of the mixture, and place it in the center of one of the egg cups. Repeat with remaining mixture. 3. Place egg cups into the air fryer basket. 4. Adjust the temperature to 320°F (160°C) and bake for 10 minutes. 5. Serve warm.
**Per Serving**
Calories: 375 | fat: 30g | protein: 23g | carbs: 3g | fiber: 0g | sodium: 445mg

## Spanish Tuna Tortilla with Roasted Peppers

**Prep time: 15 minutes | Cook time: 15 minutes | Serves 4**
6 large eggs
¼ cup (63 ml) olive oil
2 small russet potatoes, diced
1 small onion, chopped
1 roasted red bell pepper, sliced
1 (7-ounce / 198-g) can tuna packed in water, drained well and flaked
2 plum tomatoes, seeded and diced
1 teaspoon (1 g) dried tarragon

1. Preheat the broiler on high. 2. Crack the eggs in a large bowl and whisk them together until just combined. Heat the olive oil in a large, oven-safe, nonstick or cast-iron skillet over medium-low heat. 3. Add the potatoes and cook until slightly soft, about 7 minutes. Add the onion and the peppers and cook until soft, 3–5 minutes. 4. Add the tuna, tomatoes, and tarragon to the skillet and stir to combine, then add the eggs. 5. Cook for 7–10 minutes until the eggs are bubbling from the bottom and the bottom is slightly brown. 6. Place the skillet into the oven on 1 of the first 2 racks, and cook until the middle is set and the top is slightly brown. 7. Slice into wedges and serve warm or at room temperature.

**Per Serving**

Calories: 247 | fat: 14g | protein: 12g | carbs: 19g | fiber: 2g | sodium: 130mg

# Peachy Oatmeal with Pecans

**Prep time: 10 minutes | Cook time: 4 minutes | Serves 4**

4 cups (1000 ml) water

2 cups (250 g) rolled oats

1 tablespoon (15 ml) light olive oil

1 large peach, peeled, pitted, and diced

¼ teaspoon (1 g) salt

½ cup (63 g) toasted pecans

2 tablespoons (30 ml) maple syrup

1. Place water, oats, oil, peach, and salt in the Instant Pot®. Stir well. Close lid, set steam release to Sealing, press the Manual button, and set time to 4 minutes. 2. When the timer beeps, quick-release the pressure until the float valve drops. Press the Cancel button, open lid, and stir well. Serve oatmeal topped with pecans and maple syrup.

**Per Serving**

Calories: 399 | fat: 27g | protein: 8g | carbs: 35g | fiber: 7g | sodium: 148mg

# Peach Sunrise Smoothie

**Prep time: 10 minutes | Cook time: 0 minutes | Serves 1**

1 large unpeeled peach, pitted and sliced (about ½ cup)

6 ounces (170 g) vanilla or peach low-fat Greek yogurt

2 tablespoons (30 ml) low-fat milk

6 to 8 ice cubes

1. Combine all ingredients in a blender and blend until thick and creamy. Serve immediately.

**Per Serving**

Calories: 228 | fat: 3g | protein: 11g | carbs: 42g | fiber: 3g | sodium: 127mg

# Avocado Toast with Smoked Trout

**Prep time: 10 minutes | Cook time: 0 minutes | Serves 2**
1 avocado, peeled and pitted
2 teaspoons (10 ml) lemon juice, plus more for serving
¾ teaspoon ground cumin
¼ teaspoon (1 g) kosher salt
¼ teaspoon (1 g) red pepper flakes, plus more for sprinkling
¼ teaspoon (1 g) lemon zest
2 pieces whole-wheat bread, toasted
1 (3.75-ounce / 106-g) can smoked trout

1. In a medium bowl, mash together the avocado, lemon juice, cumin, salt, red pepper flakes, and lemon zest. 2. Spread half the avocado mixture on each piece of toast. Top each piece of toast with half the smoked trout. Garnish with a pinch of red pepper flakes (if desired), and/or a sprinkle of lemon juice (if desired).

**Per Serving**
Calories: 300 | fat: 20g | protein: 11g | carbs: 21g | fiber: 6g | sodium: 390mg

# Tomato and Asparagus Frittata

**Prep time: 5 minutes | Cook time: 15 minutes | Serves 4**
1 cup (250 ml) water
1 teaspoon (5 ml) olive oil
1 cup (125 g) halved cherry tomatoes
1 cup (125 g) cooked asparagus tips
¼ cup (63 g) grated Parmesan cheese
6 large eggs
¼ cup (63 g) low-fat plain Greek yogurt
½ teaspoon (3 g) salt
½ teaspoon (3 g) ground black pepper

1. Place the rack in the Instant Pot® and add water. Brush a 1.5-liter baking dish with olive oil. Add tomatoes, asparagus, and cheese to dish. 2. In a medium bowl, beat eggs, yogurt, salt, and pepper. Pour over vegetable and cheese mixture. Cover dish tightly with aluminum foil, then gently lower into machine. 3. Close lid, set steam release to Sealing, press the Manual button, and set time to 15 minutes. When the timer beeps, let pressure release naturally for 10 minutes, then quick-release any remaining pressure until the float valve drops. Press the Cancel button and open lid. Let stand for 10–15 minutes before carefully removing dish from pot. 4. Run a thin knife around the edge of the frittata and turn it out onto a serving platter. Serve warm.

**Per Serving**
Calories: 170 | fat: 11g | protein: 14g | carbs: 4g | fiber: 1g | sodium: 509mg

## Smoked Salmon Egg Scramble with Dill and Chives

**Prep time: 5 minutes | Cook time: 5 minutes | Serves 2**
4 large eggs
1 tablespoon (15 ml) milk
1 tablespoon (15 g) fresh chives, minced
1 tablespoon (15 g) fresh dill, minced
¼ teaspoon (1 g) kosher salt
⅛ teaspoon freshly ground black pepper
2 teaspoons (10 ml) extra-virgin olive oil
2 ounces (57 g) smoked salmon, thinly sliced

1. In a large bowl, whisk together the eggs, milk, chives, dill, salt, and pepper.
2. Heat the olive oil in a medium skillet or sauté pan over medium heat. Add the egg mixture and cook for about 3 minutes, stirring occasionally. 3. Add the salmon and cook until the eggs are set but moist, about 1 minute.

**Per Serving**
Calories: 325 | fat: 26g | protein: 23g | carbs: 1g | fiber: 0g | sodium: 455mg

## Marinara Eggs with Parsley

**Prep time: 5 minutes |Cook time: 15 minutes| Serves: 6**
1 tablespoon (15 ml) extra-virgin olive oil
1 cup (125 g) chopped onion (about ½ medium onion)
2 garlic cloves, minced (about 1 teaspoon / 5-g))
2 (14½-ounce / 411-g) cans Italian diced tomatoes, undrained, no salt added
6 large eggs
½ cup (30 g) chopped fresh Italian parsley
Crusty Italian bread and grated Parmesan or Romano cheese, for serving (optional)

1. In a large skillet over medium-high heat, heat the oil. Add the onion and cook for 5 minutes, stirring occasionally. Add the garlic and cook for 1 minute.
2. Pour the tomatoes with their juices over the onion mixture and cook until bubbling, 2 to 3 minutes. While waiting for the tomato mixture to bubble, crack one egg into a small custard cup or coffee mug. 3. When the tomato mixture bubbles, lower the heat to medium. Then use a large spoon to make six indentations in the tomato mixture. Gently pour the first cracked egg into one indentation and repeat, cracking the remaining eggs, one at a time, into the custard cup and pouring one into each indentation. Cover the skillet and

cook for 6 to 7 minutes, or until the eggs are done to your liking (about 6 minutes for soft-cooked, 7 minutes for harder cooked). 4. Top with the parsley, and serve with the bread and grated cheese, if desired.

**Per Serving**

Calories: 127 | fat: 7g | protein: 8g | carbs: 8g | fiber: 2g | sodium: 82mg

# Honey-Vanilla Greek Yogurt with Blueberries

**Prep time: 2 minutes| Cook time: 0 minutes | Serves 2 to3**
2 cups (500 g) plain Greek yogurt
¼ to ½ cup (62.5-125 ml) honey
¾ teaspoon vanilla extract
1 cup (125 g) blueberries

1. In a medium bowl, stir together the yogurt, honey (start with the smaller amount; you can always add more later), and vanilla. Taste and add additional honey, if needed. 2. To serve, spoon the sweetened yogurt mixture into bowls and top with the blueberries.

**Per Serving**

Calories: 295 | fat: 0g | protein: 23g | carbs: 55g | fiber: 2g | sodium: 82mg

# Power Peach Smoothie Bowl

**Prep time: 15 minutes | Cook time: 0 minutes | Serves 2**
2 cups (250 g) packed partially thawed frozen peaches
½ cup (125 g) plain or vanilla Greek yogurt
½ ripe avocado
2 tablespoons (30 g) flax meal
1 teaspoon (5 ml) vanilla extract
1 teaspoon (5 ml) orange extract
1 tablespoon (15 ml) honey (optional)

1. Combine all of the ingredients in a blender and blend until smooth. 2. Pour the mixture into two bowls, and, if desired, sprinkle with additional toppings.

**Per Serving**

Calories: 213 | fat: 13g | protein: 6g | carbs: 23g | fiber: 7g | sodium: 41mg

# Egg in a "Pepper Hole" with Avocado

**Prep time: 15 minutes | Cook time: 5 minutes | Serves 4**

4 bell peppers, any color
1 tablespoon (15 ml) extra-virgin olive oil
8 large eggs
¾ teaspoon kosher salt, divided
¼ teaspoon (1 g) freshly ground black pepper, divided
1 avocado, peeled, pitted, and diced
¼ cup (31 g) red onion, diced
¼ cup (31 g) fresh basil, chopped
Juice of ½ lime

1. Stem and seed the bell peppers. Cut 2 (2-inch-thick) rings from each pepper. Chop the remaining bell pepper into small dice, and set aside. 2. Heat the olive oil in a large skillet over medium heat. Add 4 bell pepper rings, then crack 1 egg in the middle of each ring. Season with ¼ teaspoon of the salt and ⅛ teaspoon of the black pepper. Cook until the egg whites are mostly set but the yolks are still runny, 2 to 3 minutes. Gently flip and cook 1 additional minute for over easy. Move the egg-bell pepper rings to a platter or onto plates, and repeat with the remaining 4 bell pepper rings. 3. In a medium bowl, combine the avocado, onion, basil, lime juice, reserved diced bell pepper, the remaining ¼ teaspoon kosher salt, and the remaining ⅛ teaspoon black pepper. Divide among the 4 plates.

**Per Serving** 2 egg-pepper rings:
Calories: 270 | fat: 19g | protein: 15g | carbs: 12g | fiber: 5g | sodium: 360mg

# Red Pepper and Feta Egg Bites

**Prep time: 5 minutes | Cook time: 8 minutes | Serves 6**

1 tablespoon (15 ml) olive oil
½ cup (125 g) crumbled feta cheese
¼ cup (31 g) chopped roasted red peppers
6 large eggs, beaten
¼ teaspoon (1 g) ground black pepper
1 cup (250 ml) water

1. Brush silicone muffin or poaching cups with oil. Divide feta and roasted red peppers among prepared cups. In a bowl with a pour spout, beat eggs with black pepper. 2. Place rack in the Instant Pot® and add water. Place cups on rack. Pour egg mixture into cups. Close lid, set steam release to Sealing, press the Manual button, and set time to 8 minutes. 3. When the timer beeps, quick-release the pressure until the float valve drops and open lid. Remove

silicone cups carefully and slide eggs from cups onto plates. Serve warm.

**Per Serving**

Calories: 145 | fat: 11g | protein: 10g | carbs: 3g | fiber: 1g | sodium: 294mg

# Veggie Frittata

**Prep time: 7 minutes | Cook time: 21 to 23 minutes | Serves 2**

Avocado oil spray

¼ cup (31 g) diced red onion

¼ cup (31 g) diced red bell pepper

¼ cup (31 g) finely chopped broccoli

4 large eggs

3 ounces (85 g) shredded sharp Cheddar cheese, divided

½ teaspoon (3 g) dried thyme

Sea salt and freshly ground black pepper, to taste

1. Spray a pan well with oil. Put the onion, pepper, and broccoli in the pan, place the pan in the air fryer, and set to 350°F (177°C). Bake for 5 minutes. 2. While the vegetables cook, beat the eggs in a medium bowl. Stir in half of the cheese, and season with the thyme, salt, and pepper. 3. Add the eggs to the pan and top with the remaining cheese. Set the air fryer to 350°F (177°C). Bake for 16 to 18 minutes, until cooked through.

**Per Serving**

Calories: 326 | fat: 23g | protein: 24g | carbs: 4g | fiber: 1g | sodium: 156mg

# Breakfast Hash

**Prep time: 10 minutes | Cook time: 30 minutes | Serves 6**
Oil, for spraying
3 medium russet potatoes, diced
½ yellow onion, diced
1 green bell pepper, seeded and diced
2 tablespoons (30 ml) olive oil
2 teaspoons (10 g) granulated garlic
1 teaspoon (5 g) salt
½ teaspoon (3 g) freshly ground black pepper

1. Line the air fryer basket with parchment and spray lightly with oil. 2. In a large bowl, mix together the potatoes, onion, bell pepper, and olive oil. 3. Add the garlic, salt, and black pepper and stir until evenly coated. 4. Transfer the mixture to the prepared basket. 5. Air fry at 400°F (204°C) for 20 to 30 minutes, shaking or stirring every 10 minutes, until browned and crispy. If you spray the potatoes with a little oil each time you stir, they will get even crispier.

**Per Serving**
Calories: 133 | fat: 5g | protein: 3g | carbs: 21g | fiber: 2g | sodium: 395mg

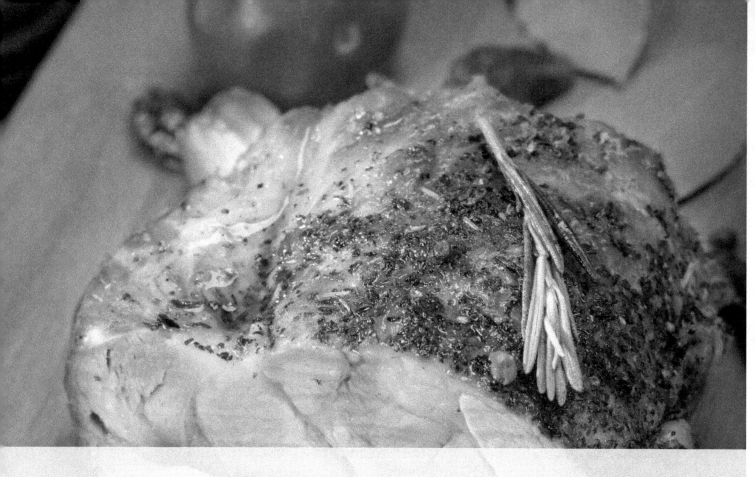

# CHAPTER 6: BEEF, PORK, AND LAMB

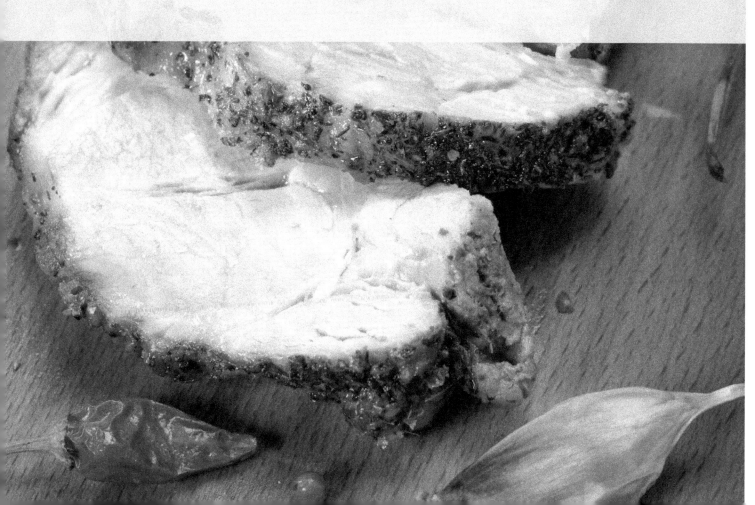

# Chapter 6: Beef, Pork, And Lamb

## Flank Steak and Blue Cheese Wraps

**Prep time: 20 minutes | Cook time: 0 minutes | Serves 6**
1 cup (125 g) leftover flank steak, cut into 1-inch slices
¼ cup (31 g) red onion, thinly sliced
¼ cup (31 g) cherry tomatoes, chopped
¼ cup (31 g) low-salt olives, pitted and chopped
¼ cup (31 g) roasted red bell peppers, drained and coarsely chopped
¼ cup (31 g) blue cheese crumbles
6 whole-wheat or spinach wraps
Sea salt and freshly ground pepper, to taste

1. Combine the flank steak, onion, tomatoes, olives, bell pepper, and blue cheese in a small bowl. 2. Spread ½ cup of this mixture on each wrap, and roll halfway. Fold the end in, and finish rolling like a burrito. 3. Cut on a diagonal if you'd like, season to taste, and serve.
**Per Serving**
Calories: 370 | fat: 26g | protein: 31g | carbs: 1g | fiber: 0g | sodium: 81mg

## Meatballs in Creamy Almond Sauce

**Prep time: 15 minutes | Cook time: 35 minutes | Serves 4 to 6**
8 ounces (227 g) ground veal or pork
8 ounces (227 g) ground beef
½ cup (63 g) finely minced onion, divided
1 large egg, beaten
¼ cup (31 g) almond flour
1½ teaspoons (7.5 g) salt, divided
1 teaspoon (5 g) garlic powder
½ teaspoon (3 g) freshly ground black pepper
½ teaspoon (3 g) ground nutmeg
2 teaspoons (10 g) chopped fresh Italian parsley, plus ¼ cup, divided
½ cup (125 ml) extra-virgin olive oil, divided
¼ cup (31 g) slivered almonds
1 cup (250 ml) dry white wine or chicken broth
¼ cup (31 g) unsweetened almond butter

1. In a large bowl, combine the veal, beef, ¼ cup onion, and the egg and mix well with a fork. In a small bowl, whisk together the almond flour, 1 teaspoon

salt, garlic powder, pepper, and nutmeg. Add to the meat mixture along with 2 teaspoons chopped parsley and incorporate well. Form the mixture into small meatballs, about 1 inch in diameter, and place on a plate. Let sit for 10 minutes at room temperature. 2. In a large skillet, heat ¼ cup oil over medium-high heat. Add the meatballs to the hot oil and brown on all sides, cooking in batches if necessary, 2 to 3 minutes per side. Remove from skillet and keep warm. 3. In the hot skillet, sauté the remaining ¼ cup minced onion in the remaining ¼ cup olive oil for 5 minutes. Reduce the heat to medium-low and add the slivered almonds. Sauté until the almonds are golden, another 3 to 5 minutes. 4. In a small bowl, whisk together the white wine, almond butter, and remaining ½ teaspoon salt. Add to the skillet and bring to a boil, stirring constantly. Reduce the heat to low, return the meatballs to skillet, and cover. Cook until the meatballs are cooked through, another 8 to 10 minutes. 5. Remove from the heat, stir in the remaining ¼ cup chopped parsley, and serve the meatballs warm and drizzled with almond sauce.

**Per Serving**

Calories: 447 | fat: 36g | protein: 20g | carbs: 7g | fiber: 2g | sodium: 659mg

# Zesty Grilled Flank Steak

**Prep time: 10 minutes | Cook time: 18 minutes | Serves 6**

¼ cup (63 ml) olive oil

3 tablespoons (45 ml) red wine vinegar

1 teaspoon (5 g) dried rosemary

1 teaspoon (5 g) dried marjoram

1 teaspoon (5 g) dried oregano

1 teaspoon (5 g) paprika

2 cloves garlic, minced

1 teaspoon (5 g) freshly ground pepper

2 pounds (907 g) flank steak

1. Combine the olive oil, vinegar, herbs, and seasonings in a small bowl. Place the flank steak in a shallow dish, and rub the marinade into the meat. Cover and refrigerate for up to 24 hours. 2. Heat a charcoal or gas grill to medium heat (375°F / 190°C). 3. Grill the steak for 18–21 minutes, turning once halfway through the cooking time. 4. An internal meat thermometer should read 140°F (60°C) when the meat is done. 5. Transfer the meat to a cutting board, and cover with aluminum foil. Let steak rest for at least 10 minutes. 6. Slice against the grain very thinly and serve.

**Per Serving**

Calories: 292 | fat: 17g | protein: 33g | carbs: 1g | fiber: 0g | sodium: 81mg

# One-Pot Pork Loin Dinner

**Prep time: 35 minutes | Cook time: 28 minutes | Serves 6**
1 tablespoon (15 ml) olive oil
1 small onion, peeled and diced
1 pound (454 g) boneless pork loin, cut into 1" pieces
½ teaspoon (3 g) salt
¼ teaspoon (1 g) ground black pepper
½ cup (125 ml) white wine
1 cup (250 ml) low-sodium chicken broth
1 large rutabaga, peeled and diced
1 large turnip, peeled and diced
4 small Yukon Gold or red potatoes, quartered
4 medium carrots, peeled and diced
1 stalk celery, finely diced
½ cup (63 g) sliced leeks, white part only
½ teaspoon (3 g) mild curry powder
¼ teaspoon (1 g) dried thyme
2 teaspoons (10 g) dried parsley
3 tablespoons (45 ml) lemon juice
2 large Granny Smith apples, peeled, cored, and diced

1. Press the Sauté button on the Instant Pot® and heat oil. Add onion and cook until tender, about 3 minutes. Add pork and season with salt and pepper. Cook until pork begins to brown, about 5 minutes. Add wine, broth, rutabaga, and turnip and stir well. Add potatoes, carrots, celery, leeks, curry powder, thyme, parsley, and lemon juice to the pot. Stir to combine. Press the Cancel button. 2. Close lid, set steam release to Sealing, press the Manual button, and set time to 15 minutes. When the timer beeps, let pressure release naturally, about 25 minutes. Press the Cancel button. 3. Open lid and add diced apples. Press the Sauté button and simmer for 5 minutes or until apples are tender. Serve immediately in large bowls.

**Per Serving**
Calories: 271 | fat: 4g | protein: 14g | carbs: 30g | fiber: 5g | sodium: 316mg

# Stuffed Pork Loin with Sun-Dried Tomato and Goat Cheese

**Prep time: 15 minutes | Cook time: 30 to 40 minutes | Serves 6**
1 to 1½ pounds (454 to 680 g) pork tenderloin
1 cup (250 g) crumbled goat cheese
4 ounces (113 g) frozen spinach, thawed and well drained
2 tablespoons (30 g) chopped sun-dried tomatoes
2 tablespoons (30 ml) extra-virgin olive oil (or seasoned oil marinade from sun-dried tomatoes), plus ¼ cup, divided
½ teaspoon (3 g) salt
½ teaspoon (3 g) freshly ground black pepper
Zucchini noodles or sautéed greens, for serving

1. Preheat the oven to 350°F(180°C). Cut cooking twine into eight (6-inch) pieces. 2. Cut the pork tenderloin in half lengthwise, leaving about an inch border, being careful to not cut all the way through to the other side. Open the tenderloin like a book to form a large rectangle. Place it between two pieces of parchment paper or plastic wrap and pound to about ¼-inch thickness with a meat mallet, rolling pin, or the back of a heavy spoon. 3. In a small bowl, combine the goat cheese, spinach, sun-dried tomatoes, 2 tablespoons olive oil, salt, and pepper and mix to incorporate well. 4. Spread the filling over the surface of the pork, leaving a 1-inch border from one long edge and both short edges. To roll, start from the long edge with filling and roll towards the opposite edge. Tie cooking twine around the pork to secure it closed, evenly spacing each of the eight pieces of twine along the length of the roll. 5. In a Dutch oven or large oven-safe skillet, heat ¼ cup olive oil over medium-high heat. Add the pork and brown on all sides. Remove from the heat, cover, and bake until the pork is cooked through, 45 to 75 minutes, depending on the thickness of the pork. Remove from the oven and let rest for 10 minutes at room temperature. 6. To serve, remove the twine and discard. Slice the pork into medallions and serve over zucchini noodles or sautéed greens, spooning the cooking oil and any bits of filling that fell out during cooking over top.
**Per Serving**
Calories: 270 | fat: 20g | protein: 20g | carbs: 2g | fiber: 1g | sodium: 392mg

# Lamb and Bean Stew

**Prep time: 15 minutes | Cook time: 35 minutes | Serves 4**
4 tablespoons (60 ml) olive oil, divided
1 pound (454 g) lamb shoulder, cut into 2-inch cubes
Sea salt
Freshly ground black pepper
2 garlic cloves, minced (optional)
1 large onion, diced
1 cup (125 g) chopped celery
1 cup (125 g) chopped tomatoes
1 cup (125 g) chopped carrots

⅓ cup tomato paste

1 (28-ounce/ 794-g) can white kidney beans, drained and rinsed
2 cups (500 ml) water

1. In a stockpot, heat 1 tablespoon of olive oil over medium-high heat. Season the lamb pieces with salt and pepper and add to the stockpot with the garlic, if desired. Brown the lamb, turning it frequently, for 3 to 4 minutes. Add the remaining 3 tablespoons of olive oil, the onion, celery, tomatoes, and carrots and cook for 4 to 5 minutes. 2. Add the tomato paste and stir to combine, then add the beans and water. Bring the mixture to a boil, reduce the heat to low, cover, and simmer for 25 minutes, or until the lamb is fully cooked. 3. Taste, adjust the seasoning, and serve.
**Per Serving**
Calories: 521 | fat: 24g | protein: 36g | carbs: 43g | fiber: 12g | sodium: 140mg

# Rosemary Pork Shoulder with Apples

**Prep time: 15 minutes | Cook time: 52 minutes | Serves 8**
1 (3½-pound / 1.6-kg) pork shoulder roast
3 tablespoons (45 g) Dijon mustard
1 tablespoon (15 ml) olive oil
½ cup (125 ml) dry white wine
2 medium tart apples, peeled, cored, and quartered
3 cloves garlic, peeled and minced
½ teaspoon (3 g) salt
½ teaspoon (3 g) ground black pepper
1 teaspoon (5 g) dried rosemary

1. Coat all sides of roast with mustard. Press the Sauté button on the Instant Pot® and heat oil. Add pork roast and brown on all sides, about 3 minutes per

side. 2. Add wine and scrape up any browned bits sticking to the bottom of the pot. Add apples, garlic, salt, pepper, and rosemary. Press the Cancel button. 3. Close lid, set steam release to Sealing, press the Manual button, and set time to 45 minutes. When the timer beeps, let pressure release naturally, about 25 minutes. 4. Open the lid. Transfer roast to a serving platter. Tent and keep warm while you use an immersion blender to purée sauce in pot. Slice roast and pour the puréed juices over the slices. Serve.

**Per Serving**

Calories: 394 | fat: 25g | protein: 33g | carbs: 5g | fiber: 1g | sodium: 393mg

# Lamb Shanks and Potatoes

**Prep time: 10 minutes | Cook time: 8 hours | Serves 6**

1(15-ounce/ 425-g) can crushed tomatoes in purée

3 tablespoons (45 g) tomato paste

2 tablespoons (30 g) apricot jam

6 cloves garlic, thinly sliced

3 strips orange zest

¾ teaspoon crushed dried rosemary

½ teaspoon (3 g) ground ginger

½ teaspoon (3 g) ground cinnamon

Coarse sea salt

Black pepper

3½ pounds (1.6 kg) lamb shanks, trimmed of excess fat and cut into 1½-inch slices

1¼ pounds (567 g) small new potatoes, halved (or quartered, if large)

1. Stir together the tomatoes and purée, tomato paste, jam, garlic, orange zest, rosemary, ginger, and cinnamon in the slow cooker. Season with salt and pepper. 2. Add the lamb and potatoes, and spoon the tomato mixture over the lamb to coat. 3. Cover and cook until the lamb and potatoes are tender, on low for 8 hours or on high for 5 hours. Season again with salt and pepper, if desired. 4. Serve hot.

**Per Serving**

Calories: 438 | fat: 10g | protein: 62g | carbs: 26g | fiber: 4g | sodium: 248mg

# Saucy Beef Fingers

**Prep time: 30 minutes | Cook time: 14 minutes | Serves 4**
1½ pounds (680 g) sirloin steak
¼ cup (63 ml) red wine
¼ cup (63 ml) fresh lime juice
1 teaspoon (5 g) garlic powder
1 teaspoon (1 g) shallot powder
1 teaspoon (5 g) celery seeds
1 teaspoon (5 g) mustard seeds
Coarse sea salt and ground black pepper, to taste
1 teaspoon (1 g) red pepper flakes
2 eggs, lightly whisked
1 cup (250 g) Parmesan cheese
1 teaspoon (1 g) paprika

1. Place the steak, red wine, lime juice, garlic powder, shallot powder, celery seeds, mustard seeds, salt, black pepper, and red pepper in a large ceramic bowl; let it marinate for 3 hours. 2. Tenderize the cube steak by pounding with a mallet; cut into 1-inch strips. 3. In a shallow bowl, whisk the eggs. In another bowl, mix the Parmesan cheese and paprika. 4. Dip the beef pieces into the whisked eggs and coat on all sides. Now, dredge the beef pieces in the Parmesan mixture. 5. Cook at 400°F (204°C) for 14 minutes, flipping halfway through the cooking time. 6. Meanwhile, make the sauce by heating the reserved marinade in a saucepan over medium heat; let it simmer until thoroughly warmed. Serve the steak fingers with the sauce on the side. Enjoy!
**Per Serving**
Calories: 483 | fat: 29g | protein: 49g | carbs: 4g | fiber: 1g | sodium: 141mg

# Braised Short Ribs with Red Wine

**Prep time: 10 minutes | Cook time: 1 hour 30 minutes to 2 hours| Serves 4**
1½ pounds (680 g) boneless beef short ribs (if using bone-in, use 3½ pounds)
1 teaspoon (5 g) salt
½ teaspoon (3 g) freshly ground black pepper
½ teaspoon (3 g) garlic powder
¼ cup (63 ml) extra-virgin olive oil
1 cup (250 ml) dry red wine (such as cabernet sauvignon or merlot)
2 to 3 cups (500-750 ml) beef broth, divided
4 sprigs rosemary

1. Preheat the oven to 350°F(180°C). 2. Season the short ribs with salt, pepper,

and garlic powder. Let sit for 10 minutes. 3. In a Dutch oven or oven-safe deep skillet, heat the olive oil over medium-high heat. 4. When the oil is very hot, add the short ribs and brown until dark in color, 2 to 3 minutes per side. Remove the meat from the oil and keep warm. 5. Add the red wine and 2 cups beef broth to the Dutch oven, whisk together, and bring to a boil. Reduce the heat to low and simmer until the liquid is reduced to about 2 cups, about 10 minutes. 6. Return the short ribs to the liquid, which should come about halfway up the meat, adding up to 1 cup of remaining broth if needed. Cover and braise until the meat is very tender, about 1½ to 2 hours. 7. Remove from the oven and let sit, covered, for 10 minutes before serving. Serve warm, drizzled with cooking liquid.

**Per Serving**

Calories: 525 | fat: 37g | protein: 34g | carbs: 5g | fiber: 1g | sodium: 720mg

# Lamb Kofte with Yogurt Sauce

**Prep time: 30 minutes | Cook time: 15 minutes | Serves 4**
1 pound (454 g) ground lamb
½ cup (10 g) finely chopped fresh mint, plus 2 tablespoons (30 g)
¼ cup (31 g) almond or coconut flour
¼ cup (31 g) finely chopped red onion
¼ cup (31 g) toasted pine nuts
2 teaspoons (10 g) ground cumin
1½ teaspoons (7.5 g) salt, divided
1 teaspoon (5 g) ground cinnamon
1 teaspoon (5 g) ground ginger
½ teaspoon (3 g) ground nutmeg
½ teaspoon (3 g) freshly ground black pepper
1 cup (250 g) plain whole-milk Greek yogurt
2 tablespoons (30 ml) extra-virgin olive oil
Zest and juice of 1 lime

1. Heat the oven broiler to the low setting. You can also bake these at high heat (450 to 475°F/ 235 to 245°C) if you happen to have a very hot broiler. Submerge four wooden skewers in water and let soak at least 10 minutes to prevent them from burning. 2. In a large bowl, combine the lamb, ½ cup mint, almond flour, red onion, pine nuts, cumin, 1 teaspoon salt, cinnamon, ginger, nutmeg, and pepper and, using your hands, incorporate all the ingredients together well. 3. Form the mixture into 12 egg-shaped patties and let sit for 10 minutes. 4. Remove the skewers from the water, thread 3 patties onto each skewer, and place on a broiling pan or wire rack on top of a baking sheet lined with aluminum foil. Broil on the top rack until golden and cooked through, 8 to 12 minutes, flipping once halfway through cooking. 5. While the meat cooks, in a small bowl, combine the yogurt, olive oil, remaining 2 tablespoons

chopped mint, remaining ½ teaspoon salt, and lime zest and juice and whisk to combine well. Keep cool until ready to use. 6. Serve the skewers with yogurt sauce.

**Per Serving**

Calories: 420 | fat: 32g | protein: 28g | carbs: 8g | fiber: 2g | sodium: 875mg

# Spiced Oven-Baked Meatballs with Tomato Sauce

**Prep time: 25 minutes | Cook time: 1 hour 5 minutes | Serves 4**

**For the Meatballs:**

1 pound (454 g) ground chuck

¼ cup (31 g) unseasoned breadcrumbs

2 garlic cloves, minced

1 teaspoon (5 g) salt

½ teaspoon (3 g) black pepper

1 teaspoon (5 g) ground cumin

3 tablespoons (3 g) chopped fresh parsley

1 egg, lightly beaten

3 tablespoons (45 ml) extra virgin olive oil

1 teaspoon (5 g) tomato paste

1 teaspoon (5 ml) red wine vinegar

2 tablespoons (30 ml) dry red wine

1 teaspoon (5 ml) fresh lemon juice

**For the sauce:**

3 medium tomatoes, chopped, or 1 (15-ounce / 425-g) can chopped tomatoes

1 tablespoon (15 g) plus 1 teaspoon tomato paste

¼ cup (63 ml) extra virgin olive oil

1 teaspoon (5 g) fine sea salt

¼ teaspoon (1 g) black pepper

¼ teaspoon (1 g) granulated sugar

1¾ cups (438 ml) hot water

1. Begin making the meatballs by combining all the ingredients in a large bowl. Knead the mixture for 3 minutes or until all the ingredients are well incorporated. Cover the bowl with plastic wrap and transfer the mixture to the refrigerator to rest for at least 20 minutes. 2. While the meatball mixture is resting, preheat the oven to 350°F (180°C) and begin making the sauce by placing all the ingredients except the hot water in a food processor. Process until smooth and then transfer the mixture to a small pan over medium heat. Add the hot water and mix well. Let the mixture come to a boil and then reduce the heat to low and simmer for 10 minutes. 3. Remove the meatball mixture from the refrigerator and shape it into 24 oblong meatballs. 4. Spread 3 tablespoons of the sauce into the bottom of a large baking dish and place the meatballs in a single layer on top of the sauce. Pour the remaining sauce over

the top of the meatballs. 5. Bake for 45 minutes or until the meatballs are lightly brown and then turn the meatballs and bake for an additional 10 minutes. (If the sauce appears to be drying out, add another ¼ cup hot water to the baking dish.) 6. Transfer the meatballs to a serving platter. Spoon the sauce over the meatballs before serving. Store covered in the refrigerator for up to 3 days or in an airtight container in the freezer for up to 3 months.

**Per Serving**

Calories: 221 | fat: 16g | protein: 14g | carbs: 5g | fiber: 1g | sodium: 661mg

# Moroccan Meatballs

**Prep time: 10 minutes |Cook time: 20 minutes| Serves: 4**

¼ cup (31 g) finely chopped onion (about ⅛ onion)

¼ cup (31 g) raisins, coarsely chopped

1 teaspoon (5 g) ground cumin

½ teaspoon (3 g) ground cinnamon

¼ teaspoon (1 g) smoked paprika

1 large egg

1 pound (454 g) ground beef (93% lean) or ground lamb

⅓ cup panko bread crumbs

1 teaspoon (5 ml) extra-virgin olive oil

1 (28-ounce/ 794-g) can low-sodium or no-salt-added crushed tomatoes

Chopped fresh mint, feta cheese, and/or fresh orange or lemon wedges, for serving (optional)

1. In a large bowl, combine the onion, raisins, cumin, cinnamon, smoked paprika, and egg. Add the ground beef and bread crumbs and mix gently with your hands. Divide the mixture into 20 even portions, then wet your hands and roll each portion into a ball. Wash your hands. 2. In a large skillet over medium-high heat, heat the oil. Add the meatballs and cook for 8 minutes, rolling around every minute or so with tongs or a fork to brown them on most sides. (They won't be cooked through.) Transfer the meatballs to a paper towel–lined plate. Drain the fat out of the pan, and carefully wipe out the hot pan with a paper towel. 3. Return the meatballs to the pan, and pour the tomatoes over the meatballs. Cover and cook on medium-high heat until the sauce begins to bubble. Lower the heat to medium, cover partially, and cook for 7 to 8 more minutes, until the meatballs are cooked through. Garnish with fresh mint, feta cheese, and/or a squeeze of citrus, if desired, and serve.

**Per Serving**

Calories: 351 | fat: 18g | protein: 28g | carbs: 23g | fiber: 5g | sodium: 170mg

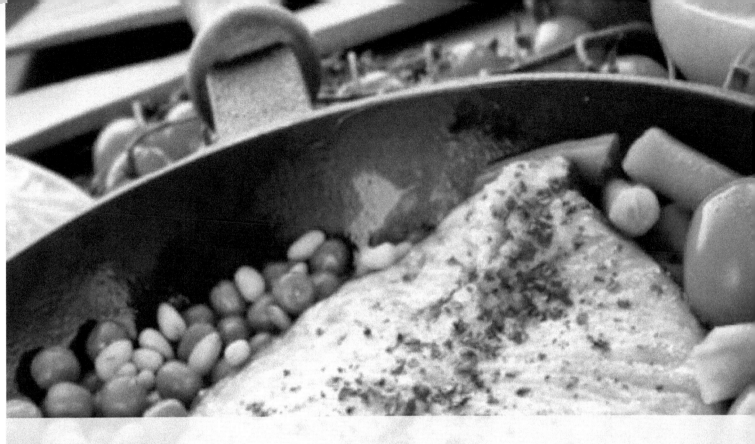

# CHAPTER 7: FISH AND SEAFOOD

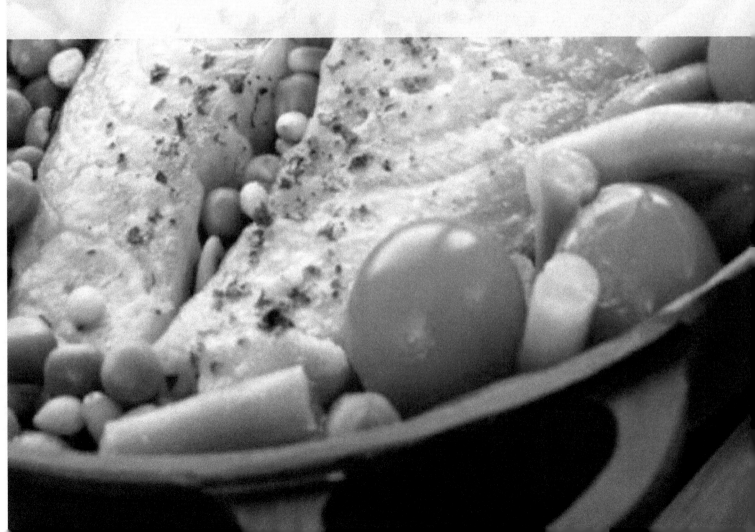

# Chapter 7: Fish And Seafood

## Cod Stew with Olives

**Prep time: 20 minutes | Cook time: 15 minutes | Serves 4**
3 tablespoons (45 ml) olive oil
1 medium onion, peeled and diced
1 stalk celery, diced
1 medium carrot, peeled and chopped
2 cloves garlic, peeled and minced
1 tablespoon (15 g) chopped fresh oregano
½ teaspoon (3 g) ground fennel seeds
1 sprig fresh thyme
1 (14½-ounce / 411-g) can diced tomatoes
1½ cup (375 ml)s vegetable broth
1 pound (454 g) cod fillets, cut into 1" pieces

⅓ cup sliced green olives

¼ teaspoon (1 g) ground black pepper
2 tablespoons (30 g) chopped dill weed

1. Press the Sauté button on the Instant Pot® and heat oil. Add onion, celery, and carrot. Cook until vegetables are soft, about 6 minutes. Add garlic, oregano, fennel seeds, and thyme. Cook for 30 seconds, then add tomatoes and vegetable broth. Stir well. Press the Cancel button. 2. Close lid, set steam release to Sealing, press the Manual button, and set time to 3 minutes. 3. When the timer beeps, quick-release the pressure until the float valve drops and open lid. Press the Cancel button, then press the Sauté button and add fish, olives, and pepper. Cook until fish is opaque, 3–5 minutes. Sprinkle with dill and serve hot.

**Per Serving**
Calories: 200 | fat: 16g | protein: 7g | carbs: 14g | fiber: 3g | sodium: 379mg

# Pistachio-Crusted Whitefish

**Prep time: 10 minutes | Cook time: 20 minutes | Serves 2**

¼ cup (31 g) shelled pistachios

1 tablespoon (15 g) fresh parsley

1 tablespoon (18 g) grated Parmesan cheese

1 tablespoon (15 g) panko bread crumbs

2 tablespoons (30 ml) olive oil

¼ teaspoon (1 g) salt

10 ounces (283 g) skinless whitefish (1 large piece or 2 smaller ones)

1. Preheat the oven to 350°F(180°C) and set the rack to the middle position. Line a sheet pan with foil or parchment paper. 2. Combine all of the ingredients except the fish in a mini food processor, and pulse until the nuts are finely ground. Alternatively, you can mince the nuts with a chef's knife and combine the ingredients by hand in a small bowl. 3. Place the fish on the sheet pan. Spread the nut mixture evenly over the fish and pat it down lightly. 4. Bake the fish for 20 to 30 minutes, depending on the thickness, until it flakes easily with a fork.

**Per Serving**

Calories: 267 | fat: 18g | protein: 28g | carbs: 1g | fiber: 0g | sodium: 85mg

# Garlicky Broiled Sardines

**Prep time: 5 minutes | Cook time: 3 minutes | Serves 4**

4 (3¼-ounce / 92-g) cans sardines (about 16 sardines), packed in water or olive oil

2 tablespoons (30 ml) extra-virgin olive oil (if sardines are packed in water)

4 garlic cloves, minced

½ teaspoon (3 g) red pepper flakes

½ teaspoon (3 g) salt

¼ teaspoon (1 g) freshly ground black pepper

1. Preheat the broiler. Line a baking dish with aluminum foil. Arrange the sardines in a single layer on the foil. 2. Combine the olive oil (if using), garlic, and red pepper flakes in a small bowl and spoon over each sardine. Season with salt and pepper. 3. Broil just until sizzling, 2 to 3 minutes. 4. To serve, place 4 sardines on each plate and top with any remaining garlic mixture that has collected in the baking dish.

**Per Serving**

Calories: 197 | fat: 11g | protein: 23g | carbs: 1g | fiber: 0g | sodium: 574mg

# Tomato-Poached Fish

**Prep time: 10 minutes | Cook time: 8 minutes | Serves 4**

2 tablespoons (30 ml) olive oil

1 medium onion, peeled and chopped

2 cloves garlic, peeled and minced

1 tablespoon (15 g) chopped fresh oregano

1 teaspoon (5 g) fresh thyme leaves

½ teaspoon (3 g) ground fennel seeds

¼ teaspoon (1 g) ground black pepper

¼ teaspoon (1 g) crushed red pepper flakes

1 (14½-ounce / 411-g) can diced tomatoes

1 cup (250 ml) vegetable broth

1 pound (454 g) halibut fillets

2 tablespoons (30 g) chopped fresh parsley

1. Press the Sauté button on the Instant Pot® and heat oil. Add onion and cook until soft, about 4 minutes. Add garlic, oregano, thyme, and fennel seeds. Cook until fragrant, about 30 seconds, then add black pepper, red pepper flakes, tomatoes, and vegetable broth. Press the Cancel button. 2. Top vegetables with fish, close lid, set steam release to Sealing, press the Manual button, and set time to 3 minutes. 3. When the timer beeps, quick-release the pressure until the float valve drops and open lid. Carefully transfer fillets to a serving platter and spoon sauce over fillets. Sprinkle with parsley and serve hot.

**Per Serving**

Calories: 212 | fat: 8g | protein: 24g | carbs: 10g | fiber: 2g | sodium: 449mg

# Shrimp over Black Bean Linguine

**Prep time: 10 minutes | Cook time: 15 minutes | Serves 4**

1 pound (454 g) black bean linguine or spaghetti

1 pound (454 g) fresh shrimp, peeled and deveined

4 tablespoons (60 ml) extra-virgin olive oil

1 onion, finely chopped

3 garlic cloves, minced

¼ cup (5 g) basil, cut into strips

1. Bring a large pot of water to a boil and cook the pasta according to the package instructions. 2. In the last 5 minutes of cooking the pasta, add the shrimp to the hot water and allow them to cook for 3 to 5 minutes. Once they turn pink, take them out of the hot water, and, if you think you may have overcooked them, run them under cool water. Set aside. 3. Reserve 1 cup of

the pasta cooking water and drain the noodles. In the same pan, heat the oil over medium-high heat and cook the onion and garlic for 7 to 10 minutes. Once the onion is translucent, add the pasta back in and toss well. 4. Plate the pasta, then top with shrimp and garnish with basil.

**Per Serving**

Calories: 668 | fat: 19g | protein: 57g | carbs: 73g | fiber: 31g | sodium: 615mg

# Italian Halibut with Grapes and Olive Oil

**Prep time: 15 minutes | Cook time: 20 minutes | Serves 4**

¼ cup (63 ml) extra-virgin olive oil

4 boneless halibut fillets, 4 ounces (113 g) each

4 cloves garlic, roughly chopped

1 small red chile pepper, finely chopped

2 cups (250 g) seedless green grapes

A handful of fresh basil leaves, roughly torn

½ teaspoon (3 g) unrefined sea salt or salt

Freshly ground black pepper

1. Heat the olive oil in a large, heavy-bottomed skillet over medium-high heat. Add the halibut, followed by the garlic, chile pepper, grapes, basil, and the salt and pepper. Pour in 1¾ cups of water, turn the heat down to medium-low, cover, and cook the fish until opaque, or for 7 minutes on each side. 2. Remove the fish from the pan and place on a large serving dish. Raise the heat, cook the sauce for 30 seconds to concentrate the flavors slightly. Taste and adjust salt and pepper. Pour sauce over the fish.

**Per Serving**

Calories: 389 | fat: 29g | protein: 17g | carbs: 15g | fiber: 1g | sodium: 384mg

# Citrus Mediterranean Salmon with Lemon Caper Sauce

**Prep time: 15 minutes | Cook time: 22 minutes | Serves 2**

2 tablespoons (30 ml) fresh lemon juice

⅓ cup orange juice

1 tablespoon (15 ml) extra virgin olive oil

⅛ teaspoon freshly ground black pepper

2 (6-ounce / 170-g) salmon fillets

Lemon Caper Sauce:

2 tablespoons (30 ml) extra virgin olive oil

1 tablespoon (15 g) finely chopped red onion

1 garlic clove, minced

2 tablespoons (30 ml) fresh lemon juice

5 ounces (142 ) dry white wine
2 tablespoons (30 g) capers, rinsed
⅛ teaspoon freshly ground black pepper

1. Preheat the oven to 350°F (180°C). 2. In a small bowl, combine the lemon juice, orange juice, olive oil, and black pepper. Whisk until blended, then pour the mixture into a zipper-lock bag. Place the fillets in the bag, shake gently, and transfer the salmon to the refrigerator to marinate for 10 minutes. 3. When the salmon is done marinating, transfer the fillets and marinade to a medium baking dish. Bake for 10–15 minutes or until the salmon is cooked through and the internal temperature reaches 165°F (74°C). Remove the salmon from the oven and cover loosely with foil. Set aside to rest. 4. While the salmon is resting, make the lemon caper sauce by heating the olive oil in a medium pan over medium heat. When the olive oil begins to shimmer, add the onions and sauté for 3 minutes, stirring frequently, then add the garlic and sauté for another 30 seconds. 5. Add the lemon juice and wine. Bring the mixture to a boil and cook until the sauce becomes thick, about 2–3 minutes, then remove the pan from the heat. Add the capers and black pepper, and stir. 6. Transfer the fillets to 2 plates, and spoon 1½ tablespoons of the sauce over each fillet. Store covered in the refrigerator for up to 3 days.
**Per Serving**
Calories: 485 | fat: 28g | protein: 36g | carbs: 11g | fiber: 1g | sodium: 331mg

# Italian Baccalà

**Prep time: 2 to 3 hours | Cook time: 4 to 6 hours | Serves 4**
1½ pounds (680 g) salt cod
1 (15-ounce / 425-g) can no-salt-added diced tomatoes
½ onion, chopped
2 garlic cloves, minced
½ teaspoon (3 g) red pepper flakes
¼ cup (5 g) chopped fresh parsley, plus more for garnish
Juice of ½ lemon

1. Wash the salt cod to remove any visible salt. Completely submerge the cod in a large bowl of water and let it soak for at least 2 to 3 hours. If you are soaking it for longer than 24 hours, change the water after 12 hours. 2. In a slow cooker, combine the tomatoes, onion, garlic, red pepper flakes, parsley, and lemon juice. Stir to mix well. Drain the cod and add it to the slow cooker, breaking it apart as necessary to make it fit. 3. Cover the cooker and cook for 4 to 6 hours on Low heat. 4. Garnish with the remaining fresh parsley for serving.
**Per Serving**
Calories: 211 | fat: 2g | protein: 39g | carbs: 8g | fiber: 2g | sodium: 179mg

# Lemon and Herb Fish Packets

**Prep time: 10 minutes | Cook time: 5 minutes | Serves 4**

1 cup (250 ml) water

4 (4-ounce / 113-g) halibut or other white fish fillets

½ teaspoon (3 g) salt

½ teaspoon (3 g) ground black pepper

1 small lemon, thinly sliced

¼ cup (5 g) chopped fresh dill

¼ cup (5 g) chopped fresh chives

2 tablespoons (30 g) chopped fresh tarragon

2 tablespoons (30 ml) extra-virgin olive oil

1. Add water to the Instant Pot® and place the rack inside. 2. Season fish fillets with salt and pepper. Measure out four pieces of foil large enough to wrap around fish fillets. Lay fish fillets on foil. Top with lemon, dill, chives, and tarragon, and drizzle each with olive oil. Carefully wrap fish loosely in foil. 3. Place packets on rack. Close lid, set steam release to Sealing, press the Steam button, and set time to 5 minutes. 4. When the timer beeps, quick-release the pressure until the float valve drops. Press the Cancel button and open lid. Serve immediately.

**Per Serving**

Calories: 185 | fat: 9g | protein: 23g | carbs: 0g | fiber: 0g | sodium: 355mg

# Tuscan Tuna and Zucchini Burgers

**Prep time: 10 minutes |Cook time: 10 minutes| Serves: 4**

3 slices whole-wheat sandwich bread, toasted

2 (5-ounce / 142-g) cans tuna in olive oil, drained

1 cup (125 g) shredded zucchini (about ¾ small zucchini)

1 large egg, lightly beaten

¼ cup (31 g) diced red bell pepper (about ¼ pepper)

1 tablespoon (15 g) dried oregano

1 teaspoon (5 g) lemon zest

¼ teaspoon (1 g) freshly ground black pepper

¼ teaspoon (1 g) kosher or sea salt

1 tablespoon (15 ml) extra-virgin olive oil

Salad greens or 4 whole-wheat rolls, for serving (optional)

1. Crumble the toast into bread crumbs using your fingers (or use a knife to cut into ¼-inch cubes) until you have 1 cup of loosely packed crumbs. Pour the crumbs into a large bowl. Add the tuna, zucchini, egg, bell pepper, oregano, lemon zest, black pepper, and salt. Mix well with a fork. With your hands,

form the mixture into four (½-cup-size) patties. Place on a plate, and press each patty flat to about ¾-inch thick. 2. In a large skillet over medium-high heat, heat the oil until it's very hot, about 2 minutes. Add the patties to the hot oil, then turn the heat down to medium. Cook the patties for 5 minutes, flip with a spatula, and cook for an additional 5 minutes. Enjoy as is or serve on salad greens or whole-wheat rolls.

**Per Serving**

Calories: 255 | fat: 11g | protein: 26g | carbs: 12g | fiber: 2g | sodium: 570mg

# Creole Crayfish

**Prep time: 10 minutes | Cook time: 3 to 4 hours | Serves 2**

1½ cups (187 g) diced celery

1 large yellow onion, chopped

2 small bell peppers, any colors, chopped

1 (8-ounce / 227-g) can tomato sauce

1 (28-ounce / 794-g) can whole tomatoes, broken up, with the juice

1 clove garlic, minced

½ teaspoon (3 g) sea salt

¼ teaspoon (1 g) black pepper

6 drops hot pepper sauce (like tabasco)

1 pound (454 g) precooked crayfish meat

1. Place the celery, onion, and bell peppers in the slow cooker. Add the tomato sauce, tomatoes, and garlic. Sprinkle with the salt and pepper and add the hot sauce. 2. Cover and cook on high for 3 to 4 hours or on low for 6 to 8 hours. 3. About 30 minutes before the cooking time is completed, add the crayfish. 4. Serve hot.

**Per Serving**

Calories: 334 | fat: 4g | protein: 43g | carbs: 34g | fiber: 13g | sodium: 659mg

# Baked Red Snapper with Potatoes and Tomatoes

**Prep time: 10 minutes | Cook time: 45 minutes | Serves 4**

5 sprigs fresh thyme, divided

2 sprigs fresh oregano, divided

1½ pounds (680 g) new potatoes, halved (or quartered if large)

4 Roma tomatoes, quartered lengthwise

1 tablespoon (15 ml) plus 1 teaspoon olive oil

4 cloves garlic, halved, divided

1¼ teaspoons (5 g) kosher salt, divided

¾ teaspoon ground black pepper, divided

1 cleaned whole red snapper (about 2 pounds / 907 g), scaled and fins

removed

½–1 lemon, sliced

4 cups (500 g) baby spinach

1. Preheat the oven to 350°F(180°C). 2. Strip the leaves off 2 sprigs thyme and 1 sprig oregano and chop. In a 9' × 13' baking dish, toss the potatoes and tomatoes with 1 tablespoon of the oil, the chopped thyme and oregano leaves, 2 cloves of the garlic, 1 teaspoon of the salt, and ½ teaspoon of the pepper. 3. Cut 3 or 4 diagonal slashes in the skin on both sides of the snapper. Rub the skin with the remaining 1 teaspoon oil. Sprinkle the cavity of the snapper with the remaining ¼ teaspoon salt and pepper. Fill it with the lemon slices, the remaining thyme and oregano sprigs, and the remaining 2 cloves garlic. Sprinkle the outside of the snapper with a pinch of salt and pepper. Set the fish on the vegetables. 4. Cover the baking dish with foil and bake for 20 minutes. Remove the foil and continue baking until the potatoes are tender and the fish flakes easily with a fork, 20 to 25 minutes. 5. Transfer the fish to a serving platter. Toss the spinach with the tomatoes and potatoes in the baking dish, until wilted. 6. Using forks, peel the skin off the fish fillets. Scatter the vegetables around the fish and serve.

**Per Serving**

Calories: 345 | fat: 6g | protein: 39g | carbs: 33g | fiber: 5g | sodium: 782mg

# Cod with Warm Beet and Arugula Salad

**Prep time: 15 minutes | Cook time: 8 minutes | Serves 4**

¼ cup (63 ml) extra-virgin olive oil, divided, plus extra for drizzling

1 shallot, sliced thin

2 garlic cloves, minced

1½ pounds (680 g) small beets, scrubbed, trimmed, and cut into ½-inch wedges

½ cup (125 ml) chicken or vegetable broth

1 tablespoon (15 g) dukkah, plus extra for sprinkling

¼ teaspoon (1 g) table salt

4 (6-ounce / 170-g) skinless cod fillets, 1½ inches thick

1 tablespoon (15 ml) lemon juice

2 ounces (57 g) baby arugula

1. Using highest sauté function, heat 1 tablespoon oil in Instant Pot until shimmering. Add shallot and cook until softened, about 2 minutes. Stir in garlic and cook until fragrant, about 30 seconds. Stir in beets and broth. Lock lid in place and close pressure release valve. Select high pressure cook function and cook for 3 minutes. Turn off Instant Pot and quick-release pressure. Carefully remove lid, allowing steam to escape away from you. 2. Fold sheet of aluminum foil into 16 by 6-inch sling. Combine 2 tablespoons oil,

dukkah, and salt in bowl, then brush cod with oil mixture. Arrange cod skinned side down in center of sling. Using sling, lower cod into Instant Pot; allow narrow edges of sling to rest along sides of insert. Lock lid in place and close pressure release valve. Select high pressure cook function and cook for 2 minutes. 3. Turn off Instant Pot and quick-release pressure. Carefully remove lid, allowing steam to escape away from you. Using sling, transfer cod to large plate. Tent with foil and let rest while finishing beet salad. 4. Combine lemon juice and remaining 1 tablespoon oil in large bowl. Using slotted spoon, transfer beets to bowl with oil mixture. Add arugula and gently toss to combine. Season with salt and pepper to taste. 5 Serve cod with salad, sprinkling individual portions with extra dukkah and drizzling with extra oil.

**Per Serving**

Calories: 340 | fat: 16g | protein: 33g | carbs: 14g | fiber: 4g | sodium: 460mg

# Italian Fish

**Prep time: 10 minutes | Cook time: 3 minutes | Serves 4**

1 (14½-ounce / 411-g) can diced tomatoes
¼ teaspoon (1 g) dried minced onion
¼ teaspoon (1 g) onion powder
¼ teaspoon (1 g) dried minced garlic
¼ teaspoon (1 g) garlic powder
¼ teaspoon (1 g) dried basil
¼ teaspoon (1 g) dried parsley
⅛ teaspoon dried oregano
¼ teaspoon (1 g) sugar
⅛ teaspoon dried lemon granules, crushed
⅛ teaspoon chili powder
⅛ teaspoon dried red pepper flakes
1 tablespoon (18 g) grated Parmesan cheese
4 (4-ounce / 113-g) cod fillets, rinsed and patted dry

1. Add tomatoes, minced onion, onion powder, minced garlic, garlic powder, basil, parsley, oregano, sugar, lemon granules, chili powder, red pepper flakes, and cheese to the Instant Pot® and stir to mix. Arrange the fillets over the tomato mixture, folding thin tail ends under to give the fillets even thickness. Spoon some of the tomato mixture over the fillets. 2. Close lid, set steam release to Sealing, press the Manual button, and set time to 3 minutes. When the timer beeps, quick-release the pressure until the float valve drops and open lid. Serve immediately.

**Per Serving**

Calories: 116 | fat: 3g | protein: 20g | carbs: 5g | fiber: 2g | sodium: 400mg

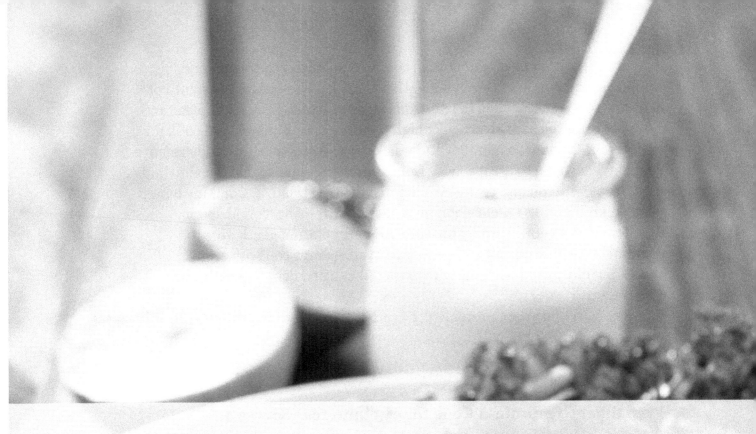

# CHAPTER 8: POULTRY

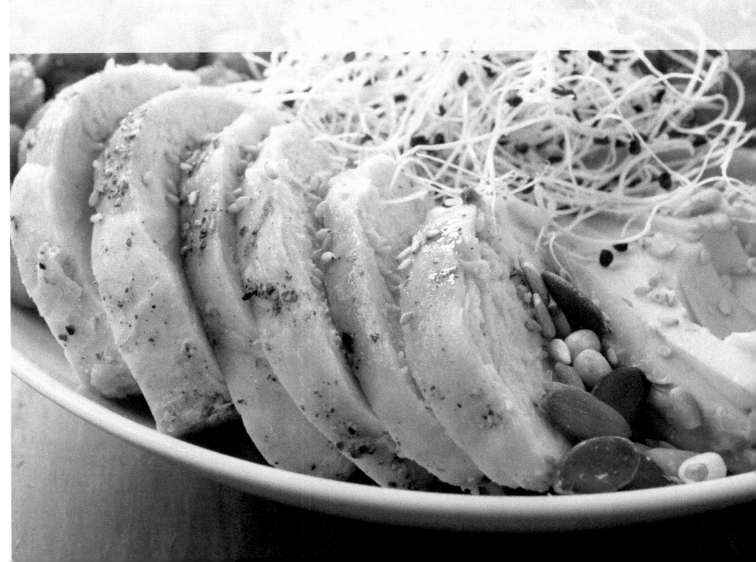

# Chapter 8: Poultry

## Whole-Roasted Spanish Chicken

**Prep time: 1 hour | Cook time: 55 minutes | Serves 4**
4 tablespoons (½ stick) unsalted butter, softened
2 tablespoons (30 g) lemon zest
2 tablespoons (30 g) smoked paprika
2 tablespoons (30 g) garlic, minced
1½ teaspoons (7.5 g) salt
1 teaspoon (5 g) freshly ground black pepper
1 (5-pound / 2.3-kg) whole chicken

1. In a small bowl, combine the butter with the lemon zest, paprika, garlic, salt, and pepper. 2. Pat the chicken dry using a paper towel. Using your hands, rub the seasoned butter all over the chicken. Refrigerate the chicken for 30 minutes. 3. Preheat the oven to 425°F(220°C). Take the chicken out of the fridge and let it sit out for 20 minutes. 4. Put the chicken in a baking dish in the oven and let it cook for 20 minutes. Turn the temperature down to 350°F (180°C) and let the chicken cook for another 35 minutes. 5. Take the chicken out of the oven and let it stand for 10 minutes before serving.
**Per Serving**
Calories: 705 | fat: 17g | protein: 126g | carbs: 4g | fiber: 1g | sodium: 880mg

## Greek Turkey Burger

**Prep time: 10 minutes | Cook time: 10 minutes | Serves 4**
1 pound (454 g) ground turkey
1 medium zucchini, grated
¼ cup (31 g) whole-wheat bread crumbs
¼ cup (31 g) red onion, minced
¼ cup (63 g) crumbled feta cheese
1 large egg, beaten
1 garlic clove, minced
1 tablespoon (15 g) fresh oregano, chopped
1 teaspoon (5 g) kosher salt
¼ teaspoon (1 g) freshly ground black pepper
1 tablespoon (15 ml) extra-virgin olive oil

1. In a large bowl, combine the turkey, zucchini, bread crumbs, onion, feta cheese, egg, garlic, oregano, salt, and black pepper, and mix well. Shape into 4

equal patties. 2. Heat the olive oil in a large nonstick grill pan or skillet over medium-high heat. Add the burgers to the pan and reduce the heat to medium. Cook on one side for 5 minutes, then flip and cook the other side for 5 minutes more.

**Per Serving**

Calories: 285 | fat: 16g | protein: 26g | carbs: 9g | fiber: 2g | sodium: 465mg

# Fiesta Chicken Plate

**Prep time: 15 minutes | Cook time: 12 to 15 minutes | Serves 4**

1 pound (454 g) boneless, skinless chicken breasts (2 large breasts)
2 tablespoons (30 ml) lime juice
1 teaspoon (5 g) cumin
½ teaspoon (3 g) salt
½ cup (125 g) grated Pepper Jack cheese
1 (16-ounce / 454-g) can refried beans
½ cup (63 g) salsa
2 cups (250 g) shredded lettuce
1 medium tomato, chopped
2 avocados, peeled and sliced
1 small onion, sliced into thin rings
Sour cream
Tortilla chips (optional)

1. Split each chicken breast in half lengthwise. 2. Mix lime juice, cumin, and salt together and brush on all surfaces of chicken breasts. 3. Place in air fryer basket and air fry at 390°F (199°C) for 12 to 15 minutes, until well done. 4. Divide the cheese evenly over chicken breasts and cook for an additional minute to melt cheese. 5. While chicken is cooking, heat refried beans on stovetop or in microwave. 6. When ready to serve, divide beans among 4 plates. Place chicken breasts on top of beans and spoon salsa over. Arrange the lettuce, tomatoes, and avocados artfully on each plate and scatter with the onion rings. 7. Pass sour cream at the table and serve with tortilla chips if desired.

**Per Serving**

Calories: 497 | fat: 27g | protein: 38g | carbs: 26g | fiber: 12g | sodium: 722mg

# Deconstructed Greek Chicken Kebabs

**Prep time: 20 minutes | Cook time: 6 to 8 hours | Serves 4**

2 pounds (907 g) boneless, skinless chicken thighs, cut into 1-inch cubes
2 zucchini (nearly 1 pound / 454 g), cut into 1-inch pieces
1 green bell pepper, seeded and cut into 1-inch pieces
1 red bell pepper, seeded and cut into 1-inch pieces
1 large red onion, chopped
2 tablespoons (30 ml) extra-virgin olive oil
2 tablespoons (30 ml) freshly squeezed lemon juice
1 tablespoon (15 ml) red wine vinegar
2 garlic cloves, minced
1 teaspoon (5 g) sea salt
1 teaspoon (5 g) dried oregano
½ teaspoon (3 g) dried basil
½ teaspoon (3 g) dried thyme
¼ teaspoon (1 g) freshly ground black pepper

1. In a slow cooker, combine the chicken, zucchini, green and red bell peppers, onion, olive oil, lemon juice, vinegar, garlic, salt, oregano, basil, thyme, and black pepper. Stir to mix well. 2. Cover the cooker and cook for 6 to 8 hours on Low heat.

**Per Serving**

Calories: 372 | fat: 17g | protein: 47g | carbs: 8g | fiber: 2g | sodium: 808mg

# Rosemary Baked Chicken Thighs

**Prep time: 20 minutes | Cook time: 20 minutes | Serves 4 to 6**

5 tablespoons (75 ml) extra-virgin olive oil, divided
3 medium shallots, diced
4 garlic cloves, peeled and crushed
1 rosemary sprig
2 to 2½ pounds (907 g to 1.1 kg) bone-in, skin-on chicken thighs (about 6 pieces)
2 teaspoons (10 g) kosher salt
¼ teaspoon (1 g) freshly ground black pepper
1 lemon, juiced and zested

⅓ cup low-sodium chicken broth

1. In a large sauté pan or skillet, heat 3 tablespoons of olive oil over medium heat. Add the shallots and garlic and cook for about a minute, until fragrant. Add the rosemary sprig. 2. Season the chicken with salt and pepper. Place it in

the skillet, skin-side down, and brown for 3 to 5 minutes. 3. Once it's cooked halfway through, turn the chicken over and add lemon juice and zest. 4. Add the chicken broth, cover the pan, and continue to cook for 10 to 15 more minutes, until cooked through and juices run clear. Serve.

**Per Serving**
Calories: 294 | fat: 18g | protein: 30g | carbs: 3g | fiber: 1g | sodium: 780mg

## Greek Yogurt–Marinated Chicken Breasts

**Prep time: 15 minutes | Cook time: 30 minutes | Serves 2**
½ cup (125 g) plain Greek yogurt
3 garlic cloves, minced
2 tablespoons (30 g) minced fresh oregano (or 1 tablespoon dried oregano)
Zest of 1 lemon
1 tablespoon (15 ml) olive oil
½ teaspoon (3 g) salt
2 (4-ounce / 113-g) boneless, skinless chicken breasts

1. In a medium bowl, add the yogurt, garlic, oregano, lemon zest, olive oil, and salt and stir to combine. If the yogurt is very thick, you may need to add a few tablespoons of water or a squeeze of lemon juice to thin it a bit. 2. Add the chicken to the bowl and toss it in the marinade to coat it well. Cover and refrigerate the chicken for at least 30 minutes or up to overnight. 3. Preheat the oven to 350°F(180°C) and set the rack to the middle position. 4. Place the chicken in a baking dish and roast for 30 minutes, or until chicken reaches an internal temperature of 165°F(74°C).

**Per Serving**
Calories: 255 | fat: 13g | protein: 29g | carbs: 8g | fiber: 2g | sodium: 694mg

## Skillet Greek Turkey and Rice

**Prep time: 20 minutes | Cook time: 30 minutes | Serves 2**
1 tablespoon (15 ml) olive oil
½ medium onion, minced
2 garlic cloves, minced
8 ounces (227 g) ground turkey breast
½ cup (63 g) roasted red peppers, chopped (about 2 jarred peppers)
¼ cup (31 g) sun-dried tomatoes, minced
1 teaspoon (5 g) dried oregano
½ cup (63 g) brown rice
1¼ cups (315 ml) low-sodium chicken stock
Salt
2 cups (250 g) lightly packed baby spinach

1. Heat the olive oil in a sauté pan over medium heat. Add the onion and sauté for 5 minutes. Add the garlic and cook for another 30 seconds. 2. Add the turkey breast and cook for 7 minutes, breaking the turkey up with a spoon, until no longer pink. 3. Add the roasted red peppers, sun-dried tomatoes, and oregano and stir to combine. Add the rice and chicken stock and bring the mixture to a boil. 4. Cover the pan and reduce the heat to medium-low. Simmer for 30 minutes, or until the rice is cooked and tender. Season with salt. 5. Add the spinach to the pan and stir until it wilts slightly.

**Per Serving**

Calories: 446 | fat: 17g | protein: 30g | carbs: 49g | fiber: 5g | sodium: 663mg

## Roasted Cornish Hen with Figs

**Prep time: 10 minutes | Cook time: 45 minutes | Serves 2**

2 Cornish game hens

2 tablespoons (30 ml) olive oil

1 tablespoon (3 g) Herbes de Provence

Sea salt and freshly ground pepper, to taste

1 pound (454 g) fresh figs

1 cup (250 ml) dry white wine

1. Preheat the oven to 350°F (180°C). 2. Place the Cornish hens in a shallow roasting pan and brush them with olive oil. 3. Season liberally with Herbes de Provence, sea salt, and freshly ground pepper. Roast the hens for 15 minutes, or until golden brown. 4. Add the figs and white wine, and cover the hens with aluminum foil. Cook an additional 20–30 minutes, or until the hens are cooked through. Allow to rest for 10 minutes before serving.

**Per Serving**

Calories: 660 | fat: 22g | protein: 50g | carbs: 48g | fiber: 7g | sodium: 166mg

## Mediterranean Roasted Turkey Breast

**Prep time: 15 minutes | Cook time: 6 to 8 hours | Serves 4**

3 garlic cloves, minced

1 teaspoon (5 g) sea salt

1 teaspoon (5 g) dried oregano

½ teaspoon (1 g) freshly ground black pepper

½ teaspoon (3 g) dried basil

½ teaspoon (3 g) dried parsley

½ teaspoon (3 g) dried rosemary

½ teaspoon (3 g) dried thyme

¼ teaspoon (1 g) dried dill weed

¼ teaspoon (1 g) ground nutmeg

2 tablespoons (30 ml) extra-virgin olive oil

2 tablespoons (30 ml) freshly squeezed lemon juice

1 (4- to 6-pound / 1.8- to 2.7-kg) boneless or bone-in turkey breast

1 onion, chopped

½ cup (125 ml) low-sodium chicken broth

4 ounces (113 g) whole Kalamata olives, pitted

1 cup (125 g) sun-dried tomatoes (packaged, not packed in oil), chopped

1. In a small bowl, stir together the garlic, salt, oregano, pepper, basil, parsley, rosemary, thyme, dill, and nutmeg. 2. Drizzle the olive oil and lemon juice all over the turkey breast and generously season it with the garlic-spice mix. 3. In a slow cooker, combine the onion and chicken broth. Place the seasoned turkey breast on top of the onion. Top the turkey with the olives and sun-dried tomatoes. 4. Cover the cooker and cook for 6 to 8 hours on Low heat. 5. Slice or shred the turkey for serving.

**Per Serving**

Calories: 676 | fat: 19g | protein: 111g | carbs: 14g | fiber: 3g | sodium: 626mg

# Herb–Marinated Chicken Breasts

**Prep time: 10 minutes | Cook time: 10 minutes | Serves 4**

½ cup (125 ml) fresh lemon juice

¼ cup (63 ml) extra-virgin olive oil

4 cloves garlic, minced

2 tablespoons (30 g) chopped fresh basil

1 tablespoon (15 g) chopped fresh oregano

1 tablespoon (15 g) chopped fresh mint

2 pounds (907 g) chicken breast tenders

½ teaspoon (3 g) unrefined sea salt or salt

¼ teaspoon (1 g) freshly ground black pepper

1. In a small bowl, whisk the lemon juice, olive oil, garlic, basil, oregano, and mint well to combine. Place the chicken breasts in a large shallow bowl or glass baking pan, and pour dressing over the top. 2. Cover, place in the refrigerator, and allow to marinate for 1 to 2 hours. Remove from the refrigerator, and season with salt and pepper. 3. Heat a large, wide skillet over medium-high heat. Using tongs, place chicken tenders evenly in the bottom of the skillet. Pour the remaining marinade over the chicken. 4. Allow to cook for 3 to 5 minutes each side, or until chicken is golden, juices have been absorbed, and meat is cooked to an internal temperature of 160°F (71°C).

**Per Serving**

Calories: 521 | fat: 35g | protein: 48g | carbs: 3g | fiber: 0g | sodium: 435mg

# Bruschetta Chicken Burgers

**Prep time: 15 minutes | Cook time: 15 minutes | Serves 2**
1 tablespoon (15 ml) olive oil
3 tablespoons (45 g) finely minced onion
2 garlic cloves, minced
1 teaspoon (5 g) dried basil
¼ teaspoon (1 g) salt
3 tablespoons (45 ml) minced sun-dried tomatoes packed in olive oil
8 ounces (227 g) ground chicken breast
3 pieces small mozzarella balls (ciliegine), minced

1. Heat the grill to high heat (about 400°F/ 205°C) and oil the grill grates. Alternatively, you can cook these in a nonstick skillet. 2. Heat the olive oil in a small skillet over medium-high heat. Add the onion and garlic and sauté for 5 minutes, until softened. Stir in the basil. Remove from the heat and place in a medium bowl. 3. Add the salt, sun-dried tomatoes, and ground chicken and stir to combine. Mix in the mozzarella balls. 4. Divide the chicken mixture in half and form into two burgers, each about ¾-inch thick. 5. Place the burgers on the grill and cook for five minutes, or until golden on the bottom. Flip the burgers over and grill for another five minutes, or until they reach an internal temperature of 165°F(74°C). 6. If cooking the burgers in a skillet on the stovetop, heat a nonstick skillet over medium-high heat and add the burgers. Cook them for 5 to 6 minutes on the first side, or until golden brown on the bottom. Flip the burgers and cook for an additional 5 minutes, or until they reach an internal temperature of 165°F(74°C).
**Per Serving**
Calories: 301 | fat: 17g | protein: 32g | carbs: 6g | fiber: 1g | sodium: 725mg

# Yogurt-Marinated Chicken Kebabs

**Prep time: 10 minutes | Cook time: 20 minutes | Serves 4**
½ cup (125 g) plain Greek yogurt
1 tablespoon (15 ml) lemon juice
½ teaspoon (3 g) ground cumin
½ teaspoon (3 g) ground coriander
½ teaspoon (3 g) kosher salt
¼ teaspoon (1 g) cayenne pepper
1½ pounds (680 g) skinless, boneless chicken breast, cut into 1-inch cubes

1. In a large bowl or zip-top bag, combine the yogurt, lemon juice, cumin, coriander, salt, and cayenne pepper. Mix together thoroughly and then add the chicken. Marinate for at least 30 minutes, and up to overnight in the

refrigerator. 2. Preheat the oven to 425°F (220°C). Line a baking sheet with parchment paper or foil. Remove the chicken from the marinade and thread it on 4 bamboo or metal skewers. 3. Bake for 20 minutes, turning the chicken over once halfway through the cooking time.

**Per Serving**

Calories: 170 | fat: 4g | protein: 31g | carbs: 1g | fiber: 0g | sodium: 390mg

# Chicken in Lemon and Herb Sauce

**Prep time: 10 minutes | Cook time: 24 minutes | Serves 4**

2 tablespoons (30 ml) olive oil

1 pound (454 g) boneless, skinless chicken breast, cut in 1" pieces

½ cup (125 ml) low-sodium chicken broth

2 tablespoons (30 ml) lemon juice

2 cloves garlic, peeled and minced

2 teaspoons (10 g) Dijon mustard

1 tablespoon (15 g) Italian seasoning

½ teaspoon (3 g) salt

1 tablespoon (15 g) grated lemon zest

¼ cup (5 g) chopped fresh parsley

1. Press the Sauté button on the Instant Pot® and heat oil. Add chicken and cook for about 4 minutes or until lightly browned on all sides. Stir in broth, lemon juice, garlic, mustard, Italian seasoning, and salt. Press the Cancel button. 2. Close lid, set steam release to Sealing, press the Poultry button, and cook for the default time of 15 minutes. When the timer beeps, let pressure release naturally for 10 minutes. Quick-release any remaining pressure until the float valve drops and then open lid. Check chicken using a meat thermometer to ensure the internal temperature is at least 165°F(74°C). Transfer chicken to a serving platter. Press the Cancel button. 3. Press the Sauté button, press the Adjust button to change the temperature to Less, and simmer uncovered for 5 minutes to thicken sauce, then pour sauce over chicken. 4. Garnish with lemon zest and chopped parsley. Serve warm.

**Per Serving**

Calories: 235 | fat: 11g | protein: 35g | carbs: 0g | fiber: 0g | sodium: 371mg

# Chicken Piccata with Mushrooms

**Prep time: 25 minutes | Cook time: 25 minutes | Serves 4**
1 pound (454 g) thinly sliced chicken breasts
1½ teaspoons (7.5 g) salt, divided
½ teaspoon (3 g) freshly ground black pepper
¼ cup (31 g) ground flaxseed
2 tablespoons (30 g) almond flour
8 tablespoons (120 ml) extra-virgin olive oil, divided
4 tablespoons (60 ml) butter, divided
2 cups (250 g) sliced mushrooms
½ cup (125 ml) dry white wine or chicken stock
¼ cup (63 ml) freshly squeezed lemon juice
¼ cup (31 g) roughly chopped capers
Zucchini noodles, for serving
¼ cup (5 g) chopped fresh flat-leaf Italian parsley, for garnish

1. Season the chicken with 1 teaspoon salt and the pepper. On a plate, combine the ground flaxseed and almond flour and dredge each chicken breast in the mixture. Set aside. 2. In a large skillet, heat 4 tablespoons olive oil and 1 tablespoon butter over medium-high heat. Working in batches if necessary, brown the chicken, 3 to 4 minutes per side. Remove from the skillet and keep warm. 3. Add the remaining 4 tablespoons olive oil and 1 tablespoon butter to the skillet along with mushrooms and sauté over medium heat until just tender, 6 to 8 minutes. 4. Add the white wine, lemon juice, capers, and remaining ½ teaspoon salt to the skillet and bring to a boil, whisking to incorporate any little browned bits that have stuck to the bottom of the skillet. Reduce the heat to low and whisk in the final 2 tablespoons butter. 5. Return the browned chicken to skillet, cover, and simmer over low heat until the chicken is cooked through and the sauce has thickened, 5 to 6 more minutes. 6. Serve chicken and mushrooms warm over zucchini noodles, spooning the mushroom sauce over top and garnishing with chopped parsley.
**Per Serving**
Calories: 596 | fat: 48g | protein: 30g | carbs: 8g | fiber: 4g | sodium: 862mg

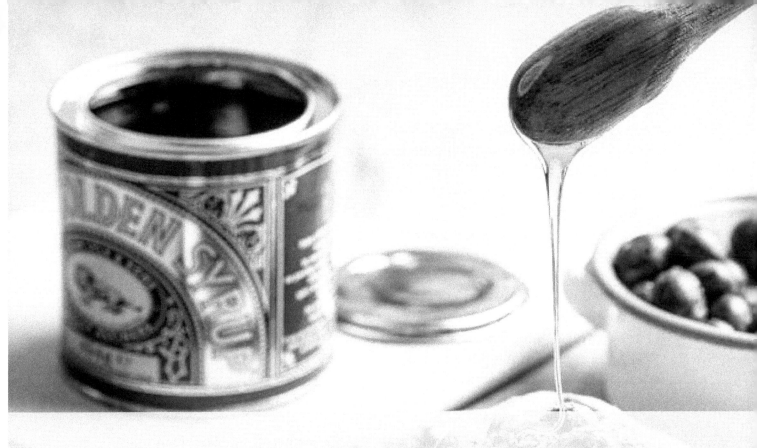

# CHAPTER 9: DESSERTS

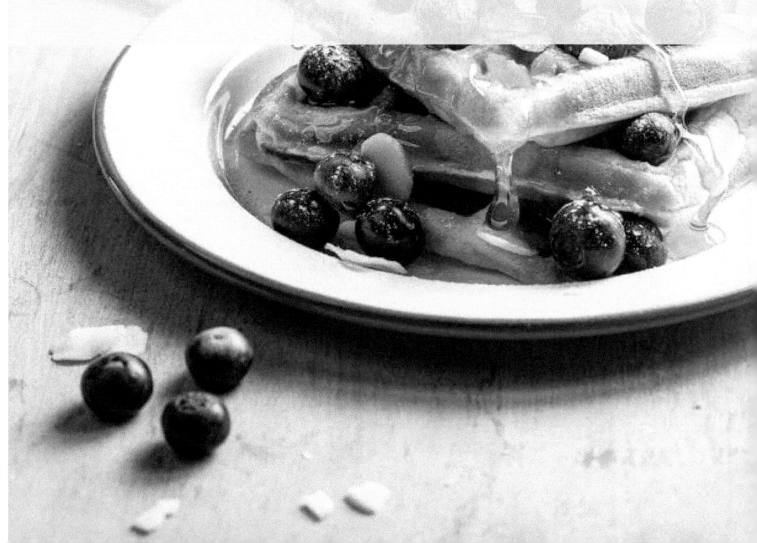

# Chapter 9: Desserts

## Fruit Compote

**Prep time: 15 minutes | Cook time: 11 minutes | Serves 6**
1 cup (250 ml) apple juice
1 cup (250 ml) dry white wine
2 tablespoons (30 ml) honey
1 cinnamon stick
¼ teaspoon (1 g) ground nutmeg
1 tablespoon (15 g) grated lemon zest
1½ tablespoons (22 g) grated orange zest
3 large apples, peeled, cored, and chopped
3 large pears, peeled, cored, and chopped
½ cup (63 g) dried cherries

1. Place all ingredients in the Instant Pot® and stir well. Close lid, set steam release to Sealing, press the Manual button, and set time to 1 minute. When the timer beeps, quick-release the pressure until the float valve drops. Press the Cancel button and open lid. 2. Use a slotted spoon to transfer fruit to a serving bowl. Remove and discard cinnamon stick. Press the Sauté button and bring juice in the pot to a boil. Cook, stirring constantly, until reduced to a syrup that will coat the back of a spoon, about 10 minutes. 3. Stir syrup into fruit mixture. Allow to cool slightly, then cover with plastic wrap and refrigerate overnight.
**Per Serving**
Calories: 211 | fat: 1g | protein: 2g | carbs: 44g | fiber: 5g | sodium: 7mg

## Spanish Cream

**Prep time: 5 minutes | Cook time: 0 minutes | Serves 6**
3 large eggs
1¼ cups (315 ml) unsweetened almond milk, divided
1 tablespoon (15 g) gelatin powder
1¼ cups (313 g) goat's cream, heavy whipping cream, or coconut cream
1 teaspoon (5 ml) vanilla powder or 1 tablespoon (15 ml) unsweetened vanilla extract
1 teaspoon (5 g) cinnamon, plus more for dusting
½ ounce (14 g) grated 100% chocolate, for topping
Optional: low-carb sweetener, to taste

1. Separate the egg whites from the egg yolks. Place ½ cup (120 ml) of the almond milk in a small bowl, then add the gelatin and let it bloom. 2. Place the yolks, cream, and the remaining ¾ cup (180 ml) almond milk in a heatproof bowl placed over a small saucepan filled with 1 cup (240 ml) of water, placed over medium heat, ensuring that the bottom of the bowl doesn't touch the water. Whisk while heating until the mixture is smooth and thickened. 3. Stir in the vanilla, cinnamon, sweetener (if using), and the bloomed gelatin. Cover with plastic wrap pressed to the surface, and chill for 30 minutes. At this point the mixture will look runny. Don't panic! This is absolutely normal. It will firm up. 4. In a bowl with a hand mixer, or in a stand mixer, whisk the egg whites until stiff, then fold them through the cooled custard. Divide among six serving glasses and chill until fully set, 3 to 4 hours. Sprinkle with the grated chocolate and, optionally, add the sweetener and a dusting of cinnamon. Store covered in the refrigerator for up to 5 days.

**Per Serving**

Calories: 172 | fat: 13g | protein: 5g | carbs: 7g | fiber: 1g | sodium: 83mg

# Individual Apple Pockets

**Prep time: 5 minutes | Cook time: 15 minutes | Serves 6**

1 organic puff pastry, rolled out, at room temperature

1 Gala apple, peeled and sliced

¼ cup (31 g) brown sugar

⅛ teaspoon ground cinnamon

⅛ teaspoon ground cardamom

Nonstick cooking spray

Honey, for topping

1. Preheat the oven to 350°F(180°C). 2. Cut the pastry dough into 4 even discs. Peel and slice the apple. In a small bowl, toss the slices with brown sugar, cinnamon, and cardamom. 3. Spray a muffin tin very well with nonstick cooking spray. Be sure to spray only the muffin holders you plan to use. 4. Once sprayed, line the bottom of the muffin tin with the dough and place 1 or 2 broken apple slices on top. Fold the remaining dough over the apple and drizzle with honey. 5. Bake for 15 minutes or until brown and bubbly.

**Per Serving**

Calories: 250 | fat: 15g | protein: 3g | carbs: 30g | fiber: 1g | sodium: 98mg

# Pears with Blue Cheese and Walnuts

**Prep time: 10 minutes | Cook time: 0 minutes | Serves 1**

1 to 2 pears, cored and sliced into 12 slices
¼ cup (63 g) blue cheese crumbles
12 walnut halves
1 tablespoon (15 ml) honey

1. Lay the pear slices on a plate, and top with the blue cheese crumbles. Top each slice with 1 walnut, and drizzle with honey. 2. Serve and enjoy!

**Per Serving**

Calories: 420 | fat: 29g | protein: 12g | carbs: 35g | fiber: 6g | sodium: 389mg

# Ricotta-Lemon Cheesecake

**Prep time: 5 minutes | Cook time: 1 hour | Serves 8 to 10**

2 (8-ounce / 227-g) packages full-fat cream cheese
1 (16-ounce / 454-g) container full-fat ricotta cheese
1½ cup (187 g) granulated sugar
1 tablespoon (15 g) lemon zest
5 large eggs
Nonstick cooking spray

1. Preheat the oven to 350°F (180°C) . 2. Using a mixer, blend together the cream cheese and ricotta cheese. 3. Blend in the sugar and lemon zest. 4. Blend in the eggs; drop in 1 egg at a time, blend for 10 seconds, and repeat. 5. Line a 9-inch springform pan with parchment paper and nonstick spray. Wrap the bottom of the pan with foil. Pour the cheesecake batter into the pan. 6. To make a water bath, get a baking or roasting pan larger than the cheesecake

pan. Fill the roasting pan about ⅓ of the way up with warm water. Put the

cheesecake pan into the water bath. Put the whole thing in the oven and let the cheesecake bake for 1 hour. 7. After baking is complete, remove the cheesecake pan from the water bath and remove the foil. Let the cheesecake cool for 1 hour on the countertop. Then put it in the fridge to cool for at least 3 hours before serving.

**Per Serving**

Calories: 489 | fat: 31g | protein: 15g | carbs: 42g | fiber: 0g | sodium: 264mg

# Halva Protein Slices

**Prep time: 5 minutes | Cook time: 0 minutes | Serves 16**

¾ cup (187 g) tahini

⅓ cup coconut butter

¼ cup (63 ml) virgin coconut oil

1 cup (125 g) collagen powder

½ teaspoon (3 g) vanilla powder or 1½ teaspoons (7.5 ml) unsweetened vanilla extract

½ teaspoon (3 g) cinnamon

⅛ teaspoon salt

Optional: low-carb sweetener, to taste

1. To soften the tahini and the coconut butter, place them in a small saucepan over low heat with the coconut oil. Remove from the heat and set aside to cool for a few minutes. 2. Add the remaining ingredients and optional sweetener. Stir to combine, then pour the mixture into an 8 × 8–inch (20 × 20 cm) parchment-lined pan or a silicone pan, or any pan or container lined with parchment paper. Place in the fridge for at least 1 hour or until fully set. 3. Cut into 16 pieces and serve. To store, keep refrigerated for up to 2 weeks or freeze to up to 3 months.

**Per Serving**

Calories: 131 | fat: 13g | protein: 2g | carbs: 3g | fiber: 1g | sodium: 33mg

# Minty Cantaloupe Granita

**Prep time: 10 minutes | Cook time: 5 minutes | Serves 4**

½ cup plus 2 tablespoons (155 ml) honey

¼ cup (63 ml) water

2 tablespoons (30 g) fresh mint leaves, plus more for garnish

1 medium cantaloupe (about 4 pounds/ 1.8 kg) peeled, seeded, and cut into 1-inch chunks

1. In a small saucepan set over low heat, combine the honey and water and cook, stirring, until the honey has fully dissolved. Stir in the mint and remove from the heat. Set aside to cool. 2. In a food processor, process the cantaloupe until very smooth. Transfer to a medium bowl. Remove the mint leaves from the syrup and discard them. Pour the syrup into the cantaloupe purée and stir to mix. 3. Transfer the mixture into a 7-by-12-inch glass baking dish and freeze, stirring with a fork every 30 minutes, for 3 to 4 hours, until it is frozen, but still grainy. Serve chilled, scooped into glasses and garnished with mint leaves.

**Per Serving**

Calories: 174 | fat: 0g | protein: 1g | carbs: 47g | fiber: 1g | sodium: 9mg

# Pomegranate-Quinoa Dark Chocolate Bark

**Prep time: 10 minutes |Cook time: 10 minutes| Serves: 6**

Nonstick cooking spray

½ cup (63 g) uncooked tricolor or regular quinoa

½ teaspoon (3 g) kosher or sea salt

8 ounces (227 g) dark chocolate or 1 cup (125 g) dark chocolate chips

½ cup (63 g) fresh pomegranate seeds

1. In a medium saucepan coated with nonstick cooking spray over medium heat, toast the uncooked quinoa for 2 to 3 minutes, stirring frequently. Do not let the quinoa burn. Remove the pan from the stove, and mix in the salt. Set aside 2 tablespoons of the toasted quinoa to use for the topping. 2. Break the chocolate into large pieces, and put it in a gallon-size zip-top plastic bag. Using a metal ladle or a meat pounder, pound the chocolate until broken into smaller pieces. (If using chocolate chips, you can skip this step.) Dump the chocolate out of the bag into a medium, microwave-safe bowl and heat for 1 minute on high in the microwave. Stir until the chocolate is completely melted. Mix the toasted quinoa (except the topping you set aside) into the melted chocolate. 3. Line a large, rimmed baking sheet with parchment paper. Pour the chocolate mixture onto the sheet and spread it evenly until the entire pan is covered. Sprinkle the remaining 2 tablespoons of quinoa and the pomegranate seeds on top. Using a spatula or the back of a spoon, press the quinoa and the pomegranate seeds into the chocolate. 4. Freeze the mixture for 10 to 15 minutes, or until set. Remove the bark from the freezer, and break it into about 2-inch jagged pieces. Store in a sealed container or zip-top plastic bag in the refrigerator until ready to serve.

**Per Serving**

Calories: 290 | fat: 17g | protein: 5g | carbs: 29g | fiber: 6g | sodium: 202mg

# Vanilla-Poached Apricots

**Prep time: 10 minutes | Cook time: 1 minute | Serves 6**
1¼ cups (315 ml) water
¼ cup (63 ml) marsala wine
¼ cup (31 g) sugar
1 teaspoon (5 g) vanilla bean paste
8 medium apricots, sliced in half and pitted

1. Place all ingredients in the Instant Pot®. Stir to combine. Close lid, set steam release to Sealing, press the Manual button, and set time to 1 minute. 2. When the timer beeps, quick-release the pressure until the float valve drops. Press the Cancel button and open lid. Let stand for 10 minutes. Carefully remove apricots from poaching liquid with a slotted spoon. Serve warm or at room temperature.

**Per Serving**
Calories: 62 | fat: 0g | protein: 2g | carbs: 14g | fiber: 1g | sodium: 10mg

# Peaches Poached in Rose Water

**Prep time: 15 minutes | Cook time: 1 minute | Serves 6**
1 cup (250 ml) water
1 cup (250 ml) rose water
¼ cup (63 ml) wildflower honey
8 green cardamom pods, lightly crushed
1 teaspoon (5 g) vanilla bean paste
6 large yellow peaches, pitted and quartered
½ cup (63 g) chopped unsalted roasted pistachio meats

1. Add water, rose water, honey, cardamom, and vanilla to the Instant Pot®. Whisk well, then add peaches. Close lid, set steam release to Sealing, press the Manual button, and set time to 1 minute. 2. When the timer beeps, quick-release the pressure until the float valve drops. Press the Cancel button and open lid. Allow peaches to stand for 10 minutes. Carefully remove peaches from poaching liquid with a slotted spoon. 3. Slip skins from peach slices. Arrange slices on a plate and garnish with pistachios. Serve warm or at room temperature.

**Per Serving**
Calories: 145 | fat: 3g | protein: 2g | carbs: 28g | fiber: 2g | sodium: 8mg

# Greek Island Almond Cocoa Bites

**Prep time: 5 minutes | Cook time: 0 minutes | Serves 6**
½ cup (63 g) roasted, unsalted whole almonds (with skins)
3 tablespoons (45 g) granulated sugar, divided
1½ teaspoons (8 g) unsweetened cocoa powder
1¼ tablespoons (19 g) unseasoned breadcrumbs
¾ teaspoon pure vanilla extract
1½ teaspoons (8 ml) orange juice

1. Place the almonds in a food processor and process until you have a coarse ground texture. 2. In a medium bowl, combine the ground almonds, 2 tablespoons sugar, the cocoa powder, and the breadcrumbs. Mix well. 3. In a small bowl, combine the vanilla extract and orange juice. Stir and then add the mixture to the almond mixture. Mix well. 4. Measure out a teaspoon of the mixture. Squeeze the mixture with your hand to make the dough stick together, then mold the dough into a small ball. 5. Add the remaining tablespoon of the sugar to a shallow bowl. Roll the balls in the sugar until covered, then transfer the bites to an airtight container. Store covered at room temperature for up to 1 week.

**Per Serving**

Calories: 102 | fat: 6g | protein: 3g | carbs: 10g | fiber: 2g | sodium: 11mg

# Nut Butter Cup Fat Bomb

**Prep time: 5 minutes | Cook time: 0 minutes | Serves 8**
½ cup (63 g) crunchy almond butter (no sugar added)
½ cup (125 ml) light fruity extra-virgin olive oil
¼ cup (31 g) ground flaxseed
2 tablespoons (30 g) unsweetened cocoa powder
1 teaspoon (5 ml) vanilla extract
1 teaspoon (5 g) ground cinnamon (optional)
1 to 2 teaspoons (5-10 ml) sugar-free sweetener of choice (optional)

1. In a mixing bowl, combine the almond butter, olive oil, flaxseed, cocoa powder, vanilla, cinnamon (if using), and sweetener (if using) and stir well with a spatula to combine. Mixture will be a thick liquid. 2. Pour into 8 mini muffin liners and freeze until solid, at least 12 hours. Store in the freezer to maintain their shape.

**Per Serving**

Calories: 239 | fat: 24g | protein: 4g | carbs: 5g | fiber: 3g | sodium: 3mg

# Fresh Figs with Chocolate Sauce

**Prep time: 5 minutes | Cook time: 0 minutes | Serves 4**
¼ cup (63 ml) honey
2 tablespoons (30 g) cocoa powder
8 fresh figs

1. Combine the honey and cocoa powder in a small bowl, and mix well to form a syrup. 2. Cut the figs in half and place cut side up. Drizzle with the syrup and serve.

**Per Serving**
Calories: 112 | fat: 1g | protein: 1g | carbs: 30g | fiber: 3g | sodium: 3mg

# Cranberry-Orange Cheesecake Pears

**Prep time: 10 minutes | Cook time: 30 minutes | Serves 5**
5 firm pears
1 cup (250 ml) unsweetened cranberry juice
1 cup (250 ml) freshly squeezed orange juice
1 tablespoon (15 ml) pure vanilla extract
½ teaspoon (3 g) ground cinnamon
½ cup (125 g) low-fat cream cheese, softened
¼ teaspoon (1 g) ground ginger
¼ teaspoon (1 ml) almond extract
¼ cup (31 g) dried, unsweetened cranberries
¼ cup (31 g) sliced almonds, toasted

1. Peel the pears and slice off the bottoms so they sit upright. Remove the inside cores, and put the pears in a wide saucepan. 2. Add the cranberry and orange juice, as well as the vanilla and cinnamon extract. 3. Bring to a boil, and reduce to a simmer. 4. Cover and simmer on low heat for 25–30 minutes, until pears are soft but not falling apart. 5. Beat the cream cheese with the ginger and almond extract. 6. Stir the cranberries and almonds into the cream cheese mixture. 7. Once the pears have cooled, spoon the cream cheese into them. 8. Boil the remaining juices down to a syrup, and drizzle over the top of the filled pears.

**Per Serving**
Calories: 187 | fat: 6g | protein: 4g | carbs: 29g | fiber: 6g | sodium: 88mg

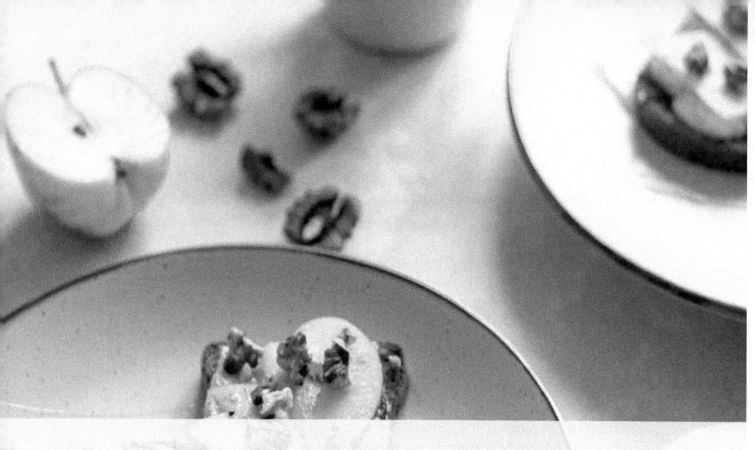

# CHAPTER 10: SNACKS AND APPETIZERS

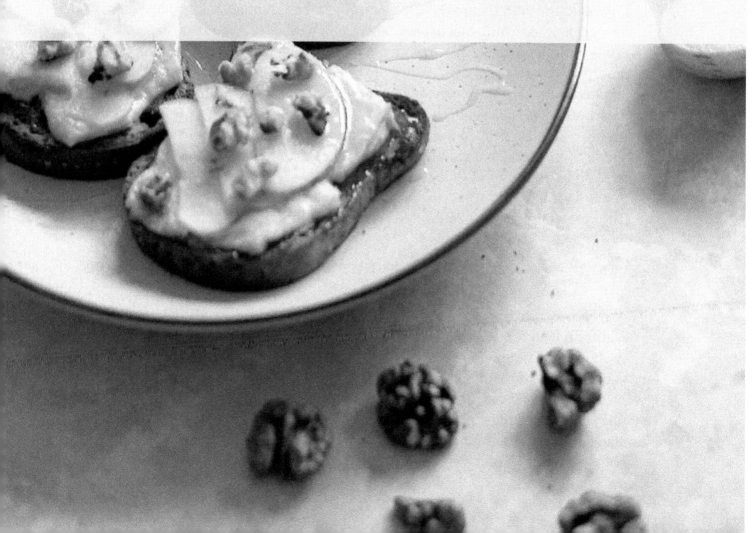

# Chapter 10: Snacks And Appetizers

## Mixed-Vegetable Caponata

**Prep time: 15 minutes | Cook time: 40 minutes | Serves 8**
1 eggplant, chopped
1 zucchini, chopped
1 red bell pepper, seeded and chopped
1 small red onion, chopped
2 tablespoons (30 ml) extra-virgin olive oil, divided
1 cup (125 g) canned tomato sauce
3 tablespoons (45 ml) red wine vinegar
1 tablespoon (15 ml) honey
¼ teaspoon (1 g) red-pepper flakes
¼ teaspoon (1 g) kosher salt
½ cup (63 g) pitted, chopped green olives
2 tablespoons (30 g) drained capers
2 tablespoons (30 g) raisins
2 tablespoons (30 g) chopped fresh flat-leaf parsley

1. Preheat the oven to 400°F(205°C). 2. On a large rimmed baking sheet, toss the eggplant, zucchini, bell pepper, and onion with 1 tablespoon of the oil. Roast until the vegetables are tender, about 30 minutes. 3. In a medium saucepan over medium heat, warm the remaining 1 tablespoon oil. Add the tomato sauce, vinegar, honey, pepper flakes, and salt and stir to combine. Add the roasted vegetables, olives, capers, raisins, and parsley and cook until bubbly and thickened, 10 minutes. 4. Remove from the heat and cool to room temperature. Serve immediately or store in an airtight container in the refrigerator for up to 1 week.
**Per Serving**
Calories: 100 | fat: 5g | protein: 2g | carbs: 13g | fiber: 4g | sodium: 464mg

## Classic Hummus with Tahini

**Prep time: 5 minutes | Cook time: 0 minutes | Makes about 2 cups**
2 cups drained canned chickpeas, liquid reserved
½ cup (125 g) tahini
¼ cup (63 ml) olive oil, plus more for garnish
2 cloves garlic, peeled, or to taste
Juice of 1 lemon, plus more as needed
1 tablespoon (15 g) ground cumin

Salt
Freshly ground black pepper
1 teaspoon (5 g) paprika, for garnish
2 tablespoons (30 g) chopped Italian parsley, for garnish
4 whole-wheat pita bread or flatbread rounds, warmed

1. In a food processor, combine the chickpeas, tahini, oil, garlic, lemon juice, and cumin. Season with salt and pepper, and process until puréed. With the food processor running, add the reserved chickpea liquid until the mixture is smooth and reaches the desired consistency. 2. Spoon the hummus into a serving bowl, drizzle with a bit of olive oil, and sprinkle with the paprika and parsley. 3. Serve immediately, with warmed pita bread or flatbread, or cover and refrigerate for up to 2 days. Bring to room temperature before serving.

**Per Serving**¼ cup:

Calories: 309 | fat: 16g | protein: 9g | carbs: 36g | fiber: 7g | sodium: 341mg

# Crispy Spiced Chickpeas

**Prep time: 5 minutes | Cook time: 25 minutes | Serves 6**
3 cans (15 ounces / 425 g each) chickpeas, drained and rinsed
1 cup (250 ml) olive oil
1 teaspoon (5 g) paprika
½ teaspoon (3 g) ground cumin
½ teaspoon (3 g) kosher salt
¼ teaspoon (1 g) ground cinnamon
¼ teaspoon (1 g) ground black pepper

1. Spread the chickpeas on paper towels and pat dry. 2. In a large saucepan over medium-high heat, warm the oil until shimmering. Add 1 chickpea; if it sizzles right away, the oil is hot enough to proceed. 3. Add enough chickpeas to form a single layer in the saucepan. Cook, occasionally gently shaking the saucepan until golden brown, about 8 minutes. With a slotted spoon, transfer to a paper towel–lined plate to drain. Repeat with the remaining chickpeas until all the chickpeas are fried. Transfer to a large bowl. 4. In a small bowl, combine the paprika, cumin, salt, cinnamon, and pepper. Sprinkle all over the fried chickpeas and toss to coat. The chickpeas will crisp as they cool.

**Per Serving**

Calories: 175 | fat: 9g | protein: 6g | carbs: 20g | fiber: 5g | sodium: 509mg

# Loaded Vegetable Pita Pizzas with Tahini Sauce

**Prep time: 5 minutes | Cook time: 12 minutes | Serves 2**

2 (6-inch) pita breads
4 canned artichoke hearts, chopped
¼ cup (31 g) chopped tomato (any variety)
¼ cup (31 g) chopped onion (any variety)
4 Kalamata olives, pitted and sliced
4 green olives, pitted and sliced
2 teaspoons (12 g) pine nuts
2 teaspoons (10 ml) extra virgin olive oil
Pinch of kosher salt
Juice of 1 lemon
**Tahini Sauce:**
2 tablespoons (36 g) tahini
2 tablespoons (30 ml) fresh lemon juice
1 tablespoon (15 ml) water
1 garlic clove, minced
Pinch of freshly ground black pepper

1. Preheat the oven to 400°F (205°C) and line a large baking sheet with wax paper. 2. Make the tahini sauce by combining the tahini and lemon juice in a small bowl. While stirring rapidly, begin adding the water, garlic, and black pepper. Continue stirring rapidly until the ingredients are well combined and smooth. 3. Place the pita breads on the prepared baking sheet. Spread about 1 tablespoon of the tahini sauce over the top of each pita and then top each pita with the chopped artichoke hearts, 2 tablespoons of the tomatoes, 2 tablespoons of the onions, half of the sliced Kalamata olives, half of the green olives, and 1 teaspoon of the pine nuts. 4. Transfer the pizzas to the oven and bake for 12 minutes or until the edges of the pita breads turn golden and crunchy. 5. Drizzle 1 teaspoon of the olive oil over each pizza, then sprinkle a pinch of kosher salt over the top followed by a squeeze of lemon. Cut the pizzas into quarters. Store covered in the refrigerator for up to 2 days.
**Per Serving**
Calories: 381 | fat: 17g | protein: 15g | carbs: 52g | fiber: 19g | sodium: 553mg

# Creamy Traditional Hummus

**Prep time: 5 minutes | Cook time: 0 minutes | Serves 8**
1 (15-ounce / 425-g) can garbanzo beans, rinsed and drained
2 cloves garlic, peeled
¼ cup (63 ml) lemon juice
1 teaspoon (5 g) salt
¼ cup (63 g) plain Greek yogurt
½ cup (125 g) tahini paste
2 tablespoons (30 ml) extra-virgin olive oil, divided

1. Add the garbanzo beans, garlic cloves, lemon juice, and salt to a food processor fitted with a chopping blade. Blend for 1 minute, until smooth. 2. Scrape down the sides of the processor. Add the Greek yogurt, tahini paste, and 1 tablespoon of olive oil and blend for another minute, until creamy and well combined. 3. Spoon the hummus into a serving bowl. Drizzle the remaining tablespoon of olive oil on top.
**Per Serving**
Calories: 189 | fat: 13g | protein: 7g | carbs: 14g | fiber: 4g | sodium: 313mg

# Mediterranean Mini Spinach Quiche

**Prep time: 15 minutes | Cook time: 25 minutes | Serves 5**
2 teaspoons (10 ml) extra virgin olive oil plus extra for greasing pan
3 eggs
3 ounces (85 g) crumbled feta
4 tablespoons (72 g) grated Parmesan cheese, divided
¼ teaspoon (1 g) freshly ground black pepper
6 ounces (170 g) frozen spinach, thawed and chopped
1 tablespoon (15 g) chopped fresh mint
1 tablespoon (15 g) chopped fresh dill

1. Preheat the oven to 375°F (190°C). Liberally grease a 10-cup muffin pan with olive oil. 2. In a medium bowl, combine the eggs, feta, 3 tablespoons of the Parmesan, black pepper, and 2 teaspoons of the olive oil. Mix well. Add the spinach, mint, and dill, and mix to combine. 3. Fill each muffin cup with 1 heaping tablespoon of the batter. Sprinkle the remaining Parmesan over the quiche. 4 Bake for 25 minutes or until the egg is set and the tops are golden. Set aside to cool for 3 minutes, then remove the quiche from the pan by running a knife around the edges of each muffin cup. Transfer the quiche to a wire rack to cool completely. 5. Store in the refrigerator for up to 3 days or freeze for up to 3 months. (If freezing, individually wrap each quiche in plastic wrap and then in foil.)

# Roasted Pepper Bruschetta with Capers and Basil

**Prep time: 10 minutes | Cook time: 15 minutes | Serves 6 to 8**

2 red bell peppers

2 yellow bell peppers

2 orange bell peppers

2 tablespoons (30 ml) olive oil, plus ¼ cup

¾ teaspoon salt, divided

½ teaspoon (3 g) freshly ground black pepper, divided

3 tablespoons (45 ml) red wine vinegar

1 teaspoon (5 g) Dijon mustard

1 clove garlic, minced

2 tablespoons (30 g) capers, drained

¼ cup (5 g) chopped fresh basil leaves, divided

1 whole-wheat baguette or other crusty bread, thinly sliced

1. Preheat the broiler to high and line a large baking sheet with aluminum foil. 2. Brush the peppers all over with 2 tablespoons of the olive oil and sprinkle with ½ teaspoon of the salt and ¼ teaspoon of the pepper. 3. Broil the peppers, turning every 3 minutes or so, until the skin is charred on all sides. Place them in a bowl, cover with plastic wrap, and let steam for 10 minutes. Slip the skins off and discard them. Seed and dice the peppers. 4. In a large bowl, whisk together the vinegar, mustard, garlic, the remaining ¼ teaspoon salt, and the remaining ¼ teaspoon of pepper. Still whisking, slowly add the remaining ¼ cup oil in a thin stream until the dressing is emulsified. Stir in the capers, 2 tablespoons of the basil, and the diced peppers. 5. Toast the bread slices and then spoon the pepper mixture over them, drizzling with extra dressing. Garnish with the remaining basil and serve immediately.

**Per Serving**

Calories: 243 | fat: 6g | protein: 8g | carbs: 39g | fiber: 4g | sodium: 755mg

# Ultimate Nut Butter

**Prep time: 5 minutes | Cook time: 30 minutes | Makes about 2 cups**

1½ cups (187 g) macadamia nuts
1 cup (125 g) pecans
½ cup (125 ml) coconut butter
5 tablespoons (90 g) light tahini
2 teaspoons (10 g) cinnamon
1 teaspoon (5 ml) vanilla powder or 1 tablespoon unsweetened vanilla extract
¼ teaspoon (1 g) salt

1. Preheat the oven to 285°F (140°C) fan assisted or 320°F (160°C) conventional. Line a baking tray with parchment. 2. Place the macadamias and pecans on the baking tray, transfer to the oven, and bake for about 30 minutes. Remove the nuts from the oven, let cool for about 10 minutes, and then transfer to a food processor while still warm. 3. Add the remaining ingredients. Blend until smooth and creamy, 2 to 3 minutes, scraping down the sides as needed with a spatula. Transfer to a jar and store at room temperature for up to 1 week or in the fridge for up to 1 month.
**Per Serving**¼ cup
Calories: 374 | fat: 39g | protein: 3g | carbs: 6g | fiber: 4g | sodium: 76mg

# Pea and Arugula Crostini with Pecorino Romano

**Prep time: 10 minutes | Cook time: 15 minutes | Serves 6 to 8**

1½ cups (187 g) fresh or frozen peas
1 loaf crusty whole-wheat bread, cut into thin slices
3 tablespoons (45 ml) olive oil, divided
1 small garlic clove, finely mined or pressed
Juice of ½ lemon
½ teaspoon (3 g) salt
¼ teaspoon (1 g) freshly ground black pepper
1 cup (60-g / packed) baby arugula
¼ cup (31 g) thinly shaved Pecorino Romano

1. Preheat the oven to 350°F(180°C). 2. Fill a small saucepan with about ½ inch of water. Bring to a boil over medium-high heat. Add the peas and cook for 3 to 5 minutes, until tender. Drain and rinse with cold water. 3. Arrange the bread slices on a large baking sheet and brush the tops with 2 tablespoons olive oil. Bake in the preheated oven for about 8 minutes, until golden brown. 4. Meanwhile, in a medium bowl, mash the peas gently with the back of a fork. They should be smashed but not mashed into a paste. Add the remaining 1 tablespoon olive oil, lemon juice, garlic, salt, and pepper and stir to mix. 5.

Spoon the pea mixture onto the toasted bread slices and top with the arugula and cheese. Serve immediately.

**Per Serving**

Calories: 301 | fat: 13g | protein: 14g | carbs: 32g | fiber: 6g | sodium: 833mg

# Croatian Red Pepper Dip

**Prep time: 10 minutes | Cook time: 30 minutes | Serves 4 to 6**

4 or 5 medium red bell peppers
1 medium eggplant (about ¾ pound / 340 g)
¼ cup (63 ml) olive oil, divided
1 teaspoon (5 g) salt, divided
½ teaspoon (3 g) freshly ground black pepper, divided
4 cloves garlic, minced
1 tablespoon (15 ml) white vinegar

1. Preheat the broiler to high. 2. Line a large baking sheet with aluminum foil. 3. Brush the peppers and eggplant all over with 2 tablespoons of the olive oil and sprinkle with ½ teaspoon of the salt and ¼ teaspoon of the pepper. Place the peppers and the eggplant on the prepared baking sheet and broil, turning every few minutes, until the skins are charred on all sides. The peppers will take about 10 minutes and the eggplant will take about 20 minutes. 4. When the peppers are fully charred, remove them from the baking sheet, place them in a bowl, cover with plastic wrap, and let them steam while the eggplant continues to cook. When the eggplant is fully charred and soft in the center, remove it from the oven and set aside to cool. 5. When the peppers are cool enough to handle, slip the charred skins off. Discard the charred skins. Seed the peppers and place them in a food processor. 6. Add the garlic to the food processor and pulse until the vegetables are coarsely chopped. Add the rest of the olive oil, the vinegar, and remaining ½ teaspoon of salt and process to a smooth purée. 7. Transfer the vegetable mixture to a medium saucepan and bring to a simmer over medium-high heat. Lower the heat to medium-low and let simmer, stirring occasionally, for 30 minutes. Remove from the heat and cool to room temperature. Serve at room temperature.

**Per Serving**

Calories: 144 | fat: 11g | protein: 2g | carbs: 12g | fiber: 5g | sodium: 471mg

# Salted Almonds

**Prep time: 5 minutes | Cook time: 25 minutes | Makes 1 cup**
1 cup (125 g) raw almonds
1 egg white, beaten
½ teaspoon (3 g) coarse sea salt

1. Preheat oven to 350°F (180°C). 2. Spread the almonds in an even layer on a baking sheet. Bake for 20 minutes until lightly browned and fragrant. 3. Coat the almonds with the egg white and sprinkle with the salt. Put back in the oven for about 5 minutes until they have dried. Cool completely before serving.

**Per Serving**
Calories: 211 | fat: 18g | protein: 8g | carbs: 8g | fiber: 5g | sodium: 305mg

# Fig-Pecan Energy Bites

**Prep time: 20 minutes |Cook time: 0 minutes| Serves: 6**
¾ cup diced dried figs (6 to 8)
½ cup (63 g) chopped pecans
¼ cup (31 g) rolled oats (old-fashioned or quick oats)
2 tablespoons (30 g) ground flaxseed or wheat germ (flaxseed for gluten-free)
2 tablespoons (36 g) powdered or regular peanut butter
2 tablespoons (30 ml) honey

1. In a medium bowl, mix together the figs, pecans, oats, flaxseed, and peanut butter. Drizzle with the honey, and mix everything together. A wooden spoon works well to press the figs and nuts into the honey and powdery ingredients. (If you're using regular peanut butter instead of powdered, the dough will be stickier to handle, so freeze the dough for 5 minutes before making the bites.) 2. Divide the dough evenly into four sections in the bowl. Dampen your hands with water—but don't get them too wet or the dough will stick to them. Using your hands, roll three bites out of each of the four sections of dough, making 12 total energy bites. 3. Enjoy immediately or chill in the freezer for 5 minutes to firm up the bites before serving. The bites can be stored in a sealed container in the refrigerator for up to 1 week.

**Per Serving**
Calories: 196 | fat: 10g | protein: 4g | carbs: 26g | fiber: 4g | sodium: 13mg

# Fried Baby Artichokes with Lemon-Garlic Aioli

**Prep time: 5 minutes | Cook time: 50 minutes | Serves 10**
**Artichokes:**
15 baby artichokes
½ lemon
3 cups (750 ml) olive oil
Kosher salt, to taste
**Aioli:**
1 egg
2 cloves garlic, chopped
1 tablespoon (15 ml) fresh lemon juice
½ teaspoon (3 g) Dijon mustard
½ cup (125 ml) olive oil
Kosher salt and ground black pepper, to taste

1. **Make the Artichokes:** Wash and drain the artichokes. With a paring knife, strip off the coarse outer leaves around the base and stalk, leaving the softer leaves on. Carefully peel the stalks and trim off all but 2' below the base. Slice off the top ½' of the artichokes. Cut each artichoke in half. Rub the cut surfaces with a lemon half to keep from browning. 2. In a medium saucepan fitted with a deep-fry thermometer over medium heat, warm the oil to about 280°F(138°C). Working in batches, cook the artichokes in the hot oil until tender, about 15 minutes. Using a slotted spoon, remove and drain on a paper towel–lined plate. Repeat with all the artichoke halves. 3. Increase the heat of the oil to 375°F(190°C). In batches, cook the precooked baby artichokes until browned at the edges and crisp, about 1 minute. Transfer to a paper towel–lined plate. Season with the salt to taste. Repeat with the remaining artichokes. 4. **Make the aioli:** In a blender, pulse together the egg, garlic, lemon juice, and mustard until combined. With the blender running, slowly drizzle in the oil a few drops at a time until the mixture thickens like mayonnaise, about 2 minutes. Transfer to a bowl and season to taste with the salt and pepper. 5. Serve the warm artichokes with the aioli on the side.
**Per Serving**
Calories: 236 | fat: 17g | protein: 6g | carbs: 21g | fiber: 10g | sodium: 283mg

# Citrus-Marinated Olives

**Prep time: 10 minutes | Cook time: 0 minutes | Makes 2 cups**

2 cups (250 g) mixed green olives with pits

¼ cup (63 ml) red wine vinegar

¼ cup (63 ml) extra-virgin olive oil

4 garlic cloves, finely minced

Zest and juice of 2 clementines or 1 large orange

1 teaspoon (5 g) red pepper flakes

2 bay leaves

½ teaspoon (3 g) ground cumin

½ teaspoon (3 g) ground allspice

1. In a large glass bowl or jar, combine the olives, vinegar, oil, garlic, orange zest and juice, red pepper flakes, bay leaves, cumin, and allspice and mix well. Cover and refrigerate for at least 4 hours or up to a week to allow the olives to marinate, tossing again before serving.

**Per Serving¼ cup:**

Calories: 112 | fat: 10g | protein: 1g | carbs: 5g | fiber: 2g | sodium: 248mg

# Appendix 1 Measurement Conversion Chart

## MEASUREMENT CONVERSION CHART

### VOLUME EQUIVALENTS(DRY)

| US STANDARD | METRIC (APPROXIMATE) |
|---|---|
| 1/8 teaspoon | 0.5 mL |
| 1/4 teaspoon | 1 mL |
| 1/2 teaspoon | 2 mL |
| 3/4 teaspoon | 4 mL |
| 1 teaspoon | 5 mL |
| 1 tablespoon | 15 mL |
| 1/4 cup | 59 mL |
| 1/2 cup | 118 mL |
| 3/4 cup | 177 mL |
| 1 cup | 235 mL |
| 2 cups | 475 mL |
| 3 cups | 700 mL |
| 4 cups | 1 L |

### VOLUME EQUIVALENTS(LIQUID)

| US STANDARD | US STANDARD (OUNCES) | METRIC (APPROXIMATE) |
|---|---|---|
| 2 tablespoons | 1 fl.oz. | 30 mL |
| 1/4 cup | 2 fl.oz. | 60 mL |
| 1/2 cup | 4 fl.oz. | 120 mL |
| 1 cup | 8 fl.oz. | 240 mL |
| 1 1/2 cup | 12 fl.oz. | 355 mL |
| 2 cups or 1 pint | 16 fl.oz. | 475 mL |
| 4 cups or 1 quart | 32 fl.oz. | 1 L |
| 1 gallon | 128 fl.oz. | 4 L |

### TEMPERATURES EQUIVALENTS

| FAHRENHEIT(F) | CELSIUS(C) (APPROXIMATE) |
|---|---|
| 225 °F | 107 °C |
| 250 °F | 120 °C |
| 275 °F | 135 °C |
| 300 °F | 150 °C |
| 325 °F | 160 °C |
| 350 °F | 180 °C |
| 375 °F | 190 °C |
| 400 °F | 205 °C |
| 425 °F | 220 °C |
| 450 °F | 235 °C |
| 475 °F | 245 °C |
| 500 °F | 260 °C |

### WEIGHT EQUIVALENTS

| US STANDARD | METRIC (APPROXIMATE) |
|---|---|
| 1 ounce | 28 g |
| 2 ounces | 57 g |
| 5 ounces | 142 g |
| 10 ounces | 284 g |
| 15 ounces | 425 g |
| 16 ounces (1 pound) | 455 g |
| 1.5 pounds | 680 g |
| 2 pounds | 907 g |

# Appendix 2 The Dirty Dozen and Clean Fifteen

## The Dirty Dozen and Clean Fifteen

The Environmental Working Group (EWG) is a nonprofit, nonpartisan organization dedicated to protecting human health and the environment Its mission is to empower people to live healthier lives in a healthier environment. This organization publishes an annual list of the twelve kinds of produce, in sequence, that have the highest amount of pesticide residue-the Dirty Dozen-as well as a list of the fifteen kinds ofproduce that have the least amount of pesticide residue-the Clean Fifteen.

### THE DIRTY DOZEN

- The 2016 Dirty Dozen includes the following produce. These are considered among the year's most important produce to buy organic:

| | |
|---|---|
| Strawberries | Spinach |
| Apples | Tomatoes |
| Nectarines | Bell peppers |
| Peaches | Cherry tomatoes |
| Celery | Cucumbers |
| Grapes | Kale/collard greens |
| Cherries | Hot peppers |

- *The Dirty Dozen list contains two additional itemskale/collard greens and hot peppers-because they tend to contain trace levels of highly hazardous pesticides.*

### THE CLEAN FIFTEEN

- The least critical to buy organically are the Clean Fifteen list. The following are on the 2016 list:

| | |
|---|---|
| Avocados | Papayas |
| Corn | Kiw |
| Pineapples | Eggplant |
| Cabbage | Honeydew |
| Sweet peas | Grapefruit |
| Onions | Cantaloupe |
| Asparagus | Cauliflower |
| Mangos | |

- *Some of the sweet corn sold in the United States are made from genetically engineered (GE) seedstock. Buy organic varieties of these crops to avoid GE produce.*